Walking out of the new road to conquer cancer (7) (Vol.7)

CREATE THE RESEARCH INSTITUTE OF THE ENVIRONMENTAL PROTECTION

and

CANCER PREVENTION AND CARRY OUT CANCER PREVENTION SYSTEM ENGINEERING

<u>Open a new era of cancer prevention research and cancer protection system engineering in the 21st century</u>

How to conquer cancer? How to prevent cancer?
How to do scientific pollution prevention and to treat pollution,
How to scientifically prevent cancer and to control cancer?

(Part I)

Authors: Xu Ze (China); Xu Jie (China) ; Bin Wu (America)
Translators: Bin Wu ; Lily Xu ; Zihao Xu ; Bo Wu
Editors: Bin Wu, Lily Xu, Tao Wu
Illustrators : Lily Xu, Bin Wu

authorHOUSE

AuthorHouse™
1663 Liberty Drive
Bloomington, IN 47403
www.authorhouse.com
Phone: 1 (800) 839-8640

© 2019 Xu Ze; Xu Jie; Bin Wu. All rights reserved.

No part of this book may be reproduced, stored in a retrieval system, or transmitted by any means without the written permission of the author.

Published by AuthorHouse   05/31/2019

ISBN: 978-1-7283-1408-2 (sc)
ISBN: 978-1-7283-1443-3 (e)

Library of Congress Control Number: 2019906224

Print information available on the last page.

Any people depicted in stock imagery provided by Getty Images are models, and such images are being used for illustrative purposes only.
Certain stock imagery © Getty Images.

This book is printed on acid-free paper.

Because of the dynamic nature of the Internet, any web addresses or links contained in this book may have changed since publication and may no longer be valid. The views expressed in this work are solely those of the author and do not necessarily reflect the views of the publisher, and the publisher hereby disclaims any responsibility for them.

Create the research institute of the environmental protection and cancer prevention and carry out cancer prevention system engineering

<u>Open a new era of cancer prevention research and cancer protection system engineering in the 21st century</u>

How to conquer cancer? How to prevent cancer?

(Part I)

- *Conduct cancer prevention research and look for carcinogenic factors*
- *Track the source of carcinogens or carcinogenic factors*
- *The way in which so many carcinogens or carcinogenic factors should be studied*
- *Study these sources of pollution and try to stop at the source*
- *Study these carcinogenic mechanisms and carcinogenic effects*
- *Study the preventive measures of how to reduce or stop these carcinogens*
- *Detection of sources of carcinogens or carcinogenic factors*
- *Try to stop the damage to human body caused by these carcinogenic factors*
- ***Try to stop cancer at the source.***
- ***Strive to eliminate security risks of cancer in the bud.***
- *This is a great project for the benefit of mankind*

TABLE OF CONTENTS

Introduction to this book xi
A Brief Introduction to The first Author xiii
A Brief Introduction to the Second Author.. xv
A brief introduction to the third author xvii
A Brief introduction to the illustrator and the advisor xix
The main topic to this book xxi
Acknowledgements... xxxiii

First, how to prevent cancer, I see one: 1

(1) Situation analysis 1
The incidence of cancer is rising.. 1
(2) Situation analysis 2
The incidence of cancer is related to the environment. 2
(3) Analysis of the situation 3.
It should improve external factors (external environment) and internal factors
 (internal environment) to prevention of carcinogenic factors 6
(4) Situation Analysis 4
Establishing the Environmental and Cancer Research Group 9
(5) Situation analysis 5
Relationship between environment and cancer.. 11
(6) Situation analysis 6
What are the carcinogenic factors in the environment? How to prevent it?.......... 19

Second, how to prevent cancer, I see two 38

(1) Finding problems and asking questions from follow-up results 38
(2) XZ-C proposes to conquer cancer and launch a general attack.............. 39
(3) XZ-C proposes to create the science city as the research bases of
 conquering cancer research bases 41

(4) XZ-C proposes to create the research institute of cancer prevention and the cancer prevention system engineering 42
(5) Cancer prevention research work cannot walk slowly and it should run forward and save the wounded 45
(6) The research work of how to improve the cure rate of cancer 49

Third, how to prevent cancer, I see three 58
(1) Why does it need to launch a general attack to conquer cancer? 58
(2) The disaster of cancer covers the whole world 61
(3) XZ-C proposed to establish cancer prevention research institute and cancer prevention system project 64
(4) Advocating scientific research ethics, medicine is benevolence, and setting up ethics is the first 65

Fourth, how to prevent cancer, I see four 67
(1) Why the research institute of the innovative environmental protection and cancer prevention should be built? 67
(2) How to create research institute of the innovative environmental protection and cancer prevention? 68
(3) Professor Xu Ze proposed: cancer prevention should be carried out from clothing, food, shelter and transportation, and cancer prevention should be carried out from the big environment and small environment 69

Fifth, XZ-C proposes to create the "the Research Institute of the Innovative Environmental Protection and Cancer Prevention " and carry out cancer prevention system engineering 79

XZ-C proposes to create the "Cancer Research Institute of Innovative Environmental Protection" and carry out cancer prevention system engineering

XZ-C proposes:

Dawning A type cancer prevention plan

Dawning B type cancer prevention plan

Dawning D-type cancer prevention plan

Macro, micro, ultra-micro

Sixth, Conduct research on cancer control and prevention and formulate cancer control plans and measures 89
(1) Relationship between environmental pollution and cancer 93
(2) Relationship between lifestyle and cancer 105
(3) Relationship between diet and cancer 116
(4) Personal prevention of cancer 134
(6) Census of cancer in the 21st century 150
(7) Prevention of cancer in the 21st century 151

INTRODUCTION TO THIS BOOK

Bin Wu and Lily Xu

In this book Dr. Xu Ze wrote down how to prevent cancer and try to stop cancer at the source and strive to eliminate security risks of cancer in the bud in detail. All of his wisdom comes from his hard work and years practices. Cancer prevention is the same important as the cancer treatment. Cancer prevention and treatment should be conducted at the same time and at the same level. It is very important for us to be aware of the cancer prevention. Once again the tears are full of both of my eyes, it is hard work all of day and night for all of our projects. The journey of getting all of these results is not always smooth and Science is endless.

With the science and technology development, cancer is gradually understood in depth. Many research data proved that more than 90% of cancer can be prevented. In this book, Dr. Xu Ze wrote down the plans of how to prevent cancer occurrence before cancer happen and how to prevent cancer from the daily life in detail. In China, there are many of the wisdom words such as: the topmost doctor manages the country; the middle level doctor prevents the disease or treats the diseases before it happens; the lowest doctor treats the diseases.

Prevention of cancer is very important. The essence is to implement and carry out the health work policy of "cancer prevention and anti-cancer" and "prevention-oriented". Our medical predecessors and the world's medical sages put forward "cancer prevention and anti-cancer" and "prevention-oriented". This policy is very correct. Let work hard together to conquer cancer and do the good things for our human being.

Bin Wu Lily Xu

05-26-2019

Timonium in Maryland, USA

A BRIEF INTRODUCTION TO THE FIRST AUTHOR

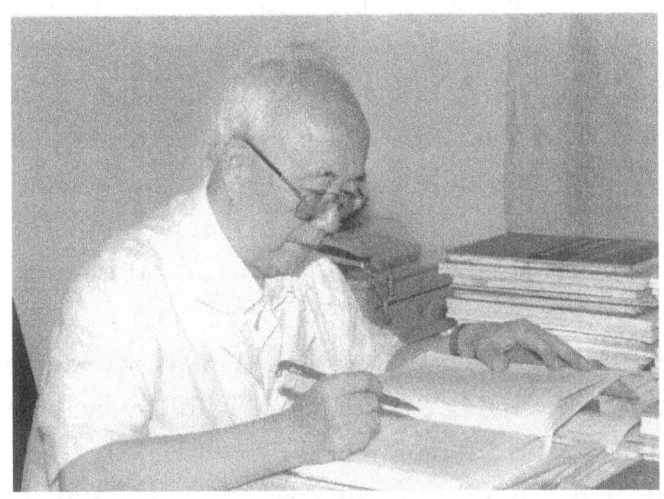

Xu Ze was born in 1933 in Leping City, Jiangxi Province, China. He graduated from Tongji Medical College in 1956. He served as the director of surgery, professor, chief physician, master and doctoral tutor of the Affiliated Hospital of Hubei College of Traditional Chinese Medicine. He is the director of the Experimental Surgery Research Institute of Hubei College of Traditional Chinese Medicine, director of the Department of Abdominal Oncology Surgery, and anti-cancer metastasis. Director of Recurrence Research Office; concurrently serves as executive director of Wuhan Branch of Chinese Medical Association, honorary president of Wuhan Anticancer Research Association, academic member of International Liver Disease Research Collaboration Center, member of International Federation of Surgeons, Chinese Journal of Experimental Surgery No. 1, 2, 3 The 4th Standing Editorial Board and the 1st, 2nd and 3rd Executive Editors of the Journal of Abdominal Surgery. He has been engaged in surgical work for 60 years and has extensive clinical experience in the surgical treatment of lung cancer, esophageal cancer, gastric cancer, liver cancer, gallbladder cancer, pancreatic cancer, and intestinal cancer, as well as the combination of Chinese and Western medicine to prevent postoperative recurrence and metastasis. In 1987, he began experimental research on tumors. Through cancer cell transplantation, he established tumor animal models, explored the mechanisms and rules of cancer metastasis and recurrence, and searched for ways to inhibit metastasis. Screening 48 kinds of natural drugs from anti-cancer invasion and metastasis And relapsed Chinese medicine, and based on this, developed xz-c immunomodulation anticancer traditional Chinese medicine preparation, clinically verified by a large number of cases, the effect is remarkable. Published 126 scientific research papers, published in 2001, "New Understanding and New Model of Cancer Treatment", published by Hubei Science and Technology Publishing House and published by Xinhua Bookstore. In 2006, he published the monograph "New Concept and New Method of Cancer Metastasis Treatment" published by Beijing People's Military Medical Publishing House and published by Xinhua Bookstore. In April 2007, he was awarded the original book award and certificate by the General Administration of Press and Publication of the People's Republic of China. In October 2011, the third monograph (New Concepts and New Methods of Cancer Treatment) was published by Beijing People's Military Medical Press. Xu Ze, Xu Jie/Zhang, Xinhua Bookstore was released. This book is translated into English by Dr. Bin Wu, published in Washington, DC on March 26, 2013, international distribution. He participated in 10 medical monographs such as "Hepatology Treatment" and "Abdominal Surgery". He engaged in teaching for 60 years, trained many young physicians, 10 master students And 2 doctoral students. He has been engaged in surgical research for 34 years and has achieved many results. Among them, "self-made xz-c: type abdominal cavity-venous bypass device for the treatment of cirrhotic refractory ascites and its clinical application" was awarded the Hubei Provincial Government Science and Technology for the second prize of the results, and promoted and applied in 38 hospitals across the country: The National Natural Science Foundation of China's experimental study on the pathophysiology and pathogenesis of pulmonary schistosomiasis by experimental surgical methods won the second prize of Hubei Provincial Government Science and Technology Achievements. He enjoys Special government allowance.

A BRIEF INTRODUCTION TO THE SECOND AUTHOR

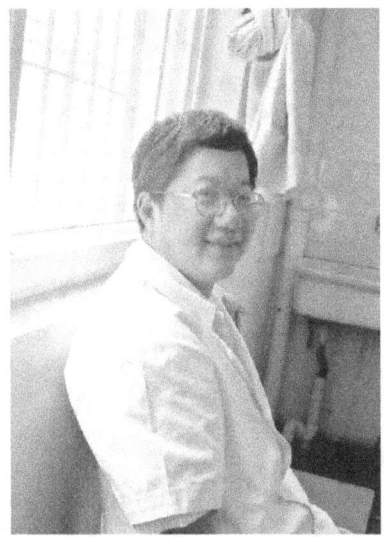

Xu Jie, male, graduated from Hubei College of Traditional Chinese Medicine in 1992, graduated from Hubei Medical University in 1996, Department of Clinical Medicine. Now He is chief physician in Hubei University of Traditional Chinese Medicine Hospital and Hubei Provincial Hospital of Surgery, engaged in experimental surgical tumor research and general surgery, urology clinical work.

Since 1992, he has been involved in the experimental tumor research of the Institute of Experimental Surgery of Hubei College of Traditional Chinese Medicine. He has carried out cancer cell transplantation and established a tumor animal model. He has carried out a series of experimental tumor research: exploring the mechanism of recurrence and metastasis of cancer and in vivo screening experiment of more than 200 kinds of Chinese herbal medicine in vivo tumor model of tumor inhibition s from a large number of natural medicine to find out, screening out of 48 kinds of anti-cancer invasion, metastasis, relapse traditional Chinese medicine

He participates in clinical validation and followed up for XZ - C immunoregulatory Chinese herbal medicine and completes the experimental research and clinical verification, data collection, collection and summary of this book.

A BRIEF INTRODUCTION TO THE THIRD AUTHOR AND THE MAIN TRANSLATOR AND THE MAIN EDITOR

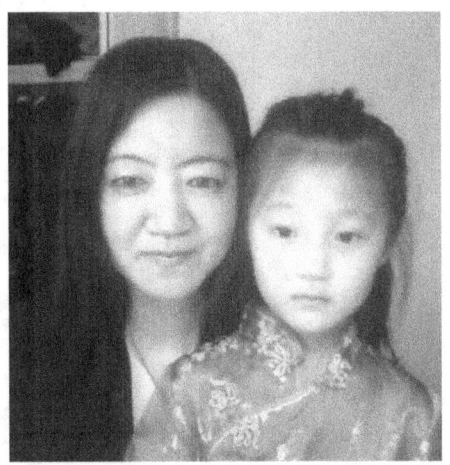

Bin Wu, MD, Ph.D., graduated from College of Yunyang of Tongji University of Medical Sciences for her MD degree; Studied her Master degree and her Ph. D degree in Sun Yat-Sen University of Medical Sciences. After she received her Ph.D., she worked as a Post-doctoral Follews in the Johns Hopkins Medical School and University of Maryland Medical School. She passed all of her USMLE tests and is going to do her residency training in America. She dedicated herself to oncology clinical and research. Her goal is to conquer cancer, which she believes this great contribution to our health. She has a daughter, named Lily Xu who drew all of the pictures in this book and is the great helper and gave the great ideas for Dr. Bin Wu.

A BRIEF INTRODUCTION TO THE ILLUSTRATOR AND THE ADVISOR

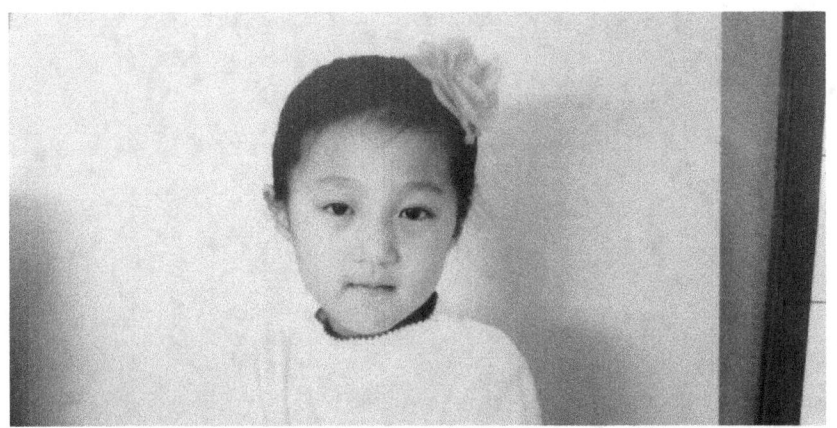

Lily Xu was born on November 17th 2006 and had an art presented in the Walter Art Museum in Baltimore at the age of 6; she got the fourth place trophy in the ES Double Digits or 24 and 24 games in the Baltimore County in Maryland; she got the first trophy in the BCPS STEM FAIR PHYSICS in Baltimore County; when she was in the sixth grade, she passed the advanced Math for 7th grade (which means the 8th grade math) test and moved the 8th grade math class and she is studying the ninth grade math; she loves the reading and writing and she finished many series of books. She got $6000 scholarship award for the Peabody music program in the Johns Hopkins University. In 2018 and 2019 she was chosen into Baltimore county Middle school Honor Band. In 2018 the robotic team which she attended for years got designing-award from the Baltimore county so that this robotic team came to Maryland State for the Robotic contest in 2019. On January 19th, 2019 she got the Robotic designing award in Maryland. She edits all of my books for the publishing and drew all of the pictures in this book. In 2019 she was chosen by Baltimore

County for one duel and one ensemble to play Clarion. In May 2019 she was award as a member of national junior honor society. In May 2019 she got an award from Maryland music association for her Clarion duel performance and an award from Maryland music association for the ensemble.

Walked out of the new road to conquer cancer (7) (Vol. 7)

THE MAIN TOPIC TO THIS BOOK

XZ-C proposes to create the research institute of the environmental protection and cancer prevention and carry out cancer prevention system engineering

Open a new era of cancer prevention research and cancer prevention system engineering in the 21st century

How to conquer cancer? How to prevent cancer?

(Part I)

- *Conduct cancer prevention research and look for carcinogenic factors*
- *Track the source of carcinogens or carcinogenic factors*
- *The way in which so many carcinogens or carcinogenic factors should be studied*
- *Study these sources of pollution and try to stop at the source*
- *Study these carcinogenic mechanisms and carcinogenic effects*
- *Study the preventive measures of how to reduce or stop these carcinogens*
- *Detection of sources of carcinogens or carcinogenic factors*
- *Try to stop the damage to human body caused by these carcinogenic factors*
- *Try to stop cancer at the source.*
- *Strive to eliminate security risks of cancer in the bud.*
- *This is a great project for the benefit of mankind*

XZ-C proposes to create the research institute of the environmental protection and cancer prevention and carry out cancer prevention system engineering

Open a new era of cancer prevention research and cancer prevention system engineering in the 21st century

- *<u>Twilight or Dawn cancer prevention A, B, D plan</u>*
- *<u>Scientific pollution prevention and pollution treatment</u>*
- *<u>Scientific cancer prevention and cancer control</u>*
- *<u>Twilight or Dawn Research Program</u>*
- *<u>Twilight or Dawn research spirit</u>*
- *<u>Medical is benevolence and to set up the moral is the first</u>*

GUIDANCE

How to conquer cancer?
How to prevent cancer by I see and how can I treat cancer by I see

XZ-C found problems and raised problems from the follow-up results (Hint: how to prevent postoperative recurrence and metastasis is the key to improve long-term outcomes after surgery)
↓
Pathfinding (to overcome cancer, where is the road? How do you find it?)
↓
Pathfinding and footprint (the series of the scientific research results and scientific and technological innovation of cancer prevention and anti-cancer metastasis research)
↓
Published cancer monographs (3 Chinese editions are exclusively distributed nationwide, 5 full English editions are published worldwide)
↓
Participated in the International Congress of Oncology (AACR Academic Conference in USA)
↓
Visiting the Stirling Cancer Institute in Houston, USA (2009)
↓
Accumulated Basic and clinical research on prevention of cancer and anti-cancer metastasis in the past more than 60 years
↓
Accumulated the clinical application experience from more than 12,000 cases in the past more than 34 years
↓
<u>**Walked Out of a new road to treat cancer with an immune regulatory and control of the combination of Chinese and Western medicine at the molecular level which are summarized the following main things:**</u>

1. <u>Walking out of a new road of cancer treatment to conquer cancer, "Chinese-style anti-cancer", Chinese and Western medicine combined with immune regulation and control</u>

2. Published the English monograph <u>"The Road to Overcome Cancer"</u> in December 6, 2016, published in USA global distribution by Author house press, INC

3. Published the English monograph <u>"Condense Wisdom and Conquer Cancer"</u> in December 2017 (Volume I), published in February 2018 (Volume II) in USA, full English version, global distribution by Author house press, Inc

4. Published the English monograph <u>"Conquer Cancer and launch The Total Attack to Cancer" – cancer prevention and cancer control and cancer treatment at the same level and at the same attention</u> published in November 2018(Volume I) in the United States by Authorhouse.com, global distribution

5. Xu Ze etc (the ninth monograph was published in the year of 87) <u>"The New progress in Cancer Treatment"</u>, published in USA in June 2018 in English, globally distributed

6. Xu Ze etc (the eleventh monograph was published in the year of 87 years old) <u>"Conquer Cancer and Launch The Total attack to Cancer"</u> in USA in November 2018 Published, full English, global distribution(Volume I)

7. Xu Ze etc(the twelfth monograph was published in the year of 88 years old) "Walked Out of the New Road to Conquer Cancer" (part I) (Volume II) in USA in January 2019 published, full English, global distribution
<u>Walked Out of the New Way of Cancer Treatment with Immune Regulation and Control of Combination of Chinese and Western Medicine(part I/ Volume 2)</u>

8. Xu Ze etc(the thirteenth monograph was published in the year of 88 years old) Walked Out of the New Road to Conquer Cancer(part II)(Volume III) in USA in January 2019 published, full English, global distribution
<u>Walked Out of the New Way of Cancer Treatment with Immune Regulation and Control of the Combination of Chinese and Western Medicine(Part II/Volume3)</u>

9. Xu Ze etc(the fourteenth monograph was published in the year of 88 years old) <u>The Research on Anticancer Traditional Chinese Medication with Immune Regulation and Control (Volume 4) in USA in February 2019 published, full English, global distribution ——Experimental Research and Clinical Application Verification</u>

10. *Xu Ze etc(the fifteenth monograph was published in the year of 88 years old)* <u>**Innovation on Clinical Application Theory of Cancer Prevention and Treatment Research in the 21st Century**</u>
 (Volume V) in USA in February 2019 published, full English, global distribution

11. *Xu Ze etc (the fifth book published at the age of 82)* <u>**"On Innovation of Treatment of Cancer"**</u>, *published in USA in December 2015, full English version, global distribution*

12. *Xu Ze, etc(fixteenth monograph was published in the year of 88 years old)* <u>**Build up the multidisciplinary and the science city of the research base with related to cancer research for conquering cancer**</u> *(Volume 6) in March 2019 full English version, global distribution*

13. <u>*Xu Ze etc*</u> *<<New understanding and new models of cancer treatment>> Contents in Chinese*

14. <u>*Xu Ze etc*</u> *<<New Concepts and New Methods for Cancer Metastasis Treatment>> in Chinese*

15. <u>*Xu Ze etc*</u> *<<New Concepts and New Methods for Cancer Treatment>> in Chinese*

The library of Prevention of Cancer and Anti-cancer medical research

The following three aspect :

1. The Collected Works of Professor Xu Ze's Research on Cancer Prevention and Cancer Treatment

XZ-C proposed: How to overcome cancer? How to prevent cancer? How to treat cancer?

<u>XZ-C new concept of cancer treatment</u>

Volume I *<<Conquer Cancer and Launch the total attack to cancer ——prevention cancer and cancer control and cancer treatment at the same level and at the same attention and at the same time>> The book table or contents or directory (omitted)*

Volume II *<<Walked out of a new way of cancer treatment with the immune regulation and control of the combination of Chinese and Western medicine>> The book table or contents or directory (omitted)*

Volume III *<<The research of XZ-C immunomodulation anticancer Chinese medicine —— Experimental research and clinical verification>> The book table or contents or directory (omitted)*

Volume IV *<<To build the multidisciplinary and the science base of cancer-related research for conquering cancer- the Science City>> Contents (omitted)*

Volume V *<<Theoretical Innovation of Cancer Prevention and Management or treatment cancer in the 21st Century>> Contents (Omitted)*

Volume VI <<*XZ-C proposes to create the preventing cancer research institute and to carry out a series of cancer prevention projects*>> Contents (Omitted)

Dawning C plan
Dawning A·B·D plan
Prevention of Cancer and Treatment of Cancer and Preventin of Cancer and anti-cancer
The Dawning Science Research Program
The Dawning Scientific research spirit
Doctor is benevolence, to set up the moral is first

Volume VII <<*Condense Wisdom and Conquer Cancer - Benefiting Mankind*>> Contents (Omitted) (Volume I and II, which book has two parts)

Volume VIII <<*The Road to Overcome Cancer*>> Directory (omitted)

Volume IX <<*On Innovation of Treatment of Cancer*>> Contents (omitted)

Volume X <<*New understanding and new models of cancer treatment*>> Contents (omitted)

Volume XI <<*New Concepts and New Methods for Cancer Metastasis Treatment*>> Table of Contents (omitted)

Volume XII <<*New Progress in Cancer Therapy*>> Table of Contents (omitted)

Volume XIII <<*New Concepts and New Methods for Cancer Treatment*>> Table of Contents (omitted)

[Note: Each volume is a published monograph on cancer medical research]

Note:

1. **_XZ-C is Xu Ze-China, because science is borderless, but scientists have national and intellectual property._**
2. **_Cancer is a disaster for all mankind. It must evoke the struggle of the people all over the world. Therefore, there are 8 monographs in the series, which are all in English, distributed worldwide, and published on authorhouse.com._**

How to conquer cancer? How to prevent cancer? How to treat cancer? How to overcome cancer and to launch the general attack of cancer?

2. Professor Xu Ze (XZ-C) summed up the collection, agglutinated wisdom, and proposed 1 to 8 of <u>"walk out of a new path to overcome cancer"</u> in order to help or to facilitate clinical application and to become the clinical reference.

In the past 60 years, the series of the scientific research achievements and the series of scientific and technological innovations which takes "conquer cancer" as the direction done by us are in this series of "monographs"; the following thesis or lemma are first proposed internationally, all of which are original papers, internationally pioneered, and have reached the forefront of the world.

<u>*XZ-C's scientific thinking, scientific research design, academic thinking, and scientific dedication about conquering cancer and launching the total cancer attack are summarized as the following monographs.*</u>

<u>*Professor Xu Ze (XZ-C) put forward the "new concept of cancer treatment" and published 1-8 monograph "Get out of the new road to conquer cancer":*</u>

1. "Walk out of a new road to conquer cancer" (1)　（一）
   "Conquer cancer and launch the total attack to cancer – the prevention of cancer and cancer control and cancer treatment at the same level"

2. "Walk out of a new road to conquer cancer" (2)　（二）
   "Walking out of a new way of cancer treatment with immune control and regulation of the combination of Chinese and Western medicine" (Part I), (Part 2)

3. "Walk out of a new road to conquer cancer" (3)　（三）
   "The research of XZ-C immunomodulation anticancer Chinese medicine"

——Experimental research and clinical verification

4. "Walked out of a new road to conquer cancer" (4) （四）
   **"Creating a Science City of Scientific Research Bases with Cancer Multidisciplinary and Cancer related research
   For conquering cancer"**

5. "Walked out of a new road to conquer cancer" (5) （五）
   "The Clinical Application Theory Innovation of 21st Century Cancer Prevention and Treatment Research"

6. "Walked out of a new road to conquer cancer" (6) （六）
   XZ-C proposes <<to create the Cancer Prevention Research Institute of Environmental Protection >> and to carry out the system engineering of the cancer prevention

   (1). *Prevention of Pollution and Treatment and Control of Pollution and Prevention of cancer and Anti-cancer anti-cancer*
   (2). *Dawning prevention cancer research plan and Dawning scientific research spirit*
   (3). *Medical is benevolence and set up the moral is the first*

7. "Walk out of a new road to conquer cancer" (7) （七）
   **"Condense wisdom and conquer cancer - for the benefit of mankind"
   (part 1), (part 2)**

8. "Walk out of a new road to conquer cancer" (8) （八）
   "The Road to overcome cancer"

3. The monographs on cancer research published by Professor Xu Ze (XZ-C)

Professor Xu Ze continues to do the research after he retired, and the science's journey was non-stop, continues to achieve the following series of scientific research results.

In 1996, I was 63 years old and retired. After I retired, I have been living in a small building for more than 20 years. I have been working alone and fighting alone. I have continued a series of experimental studies and clinical verification observations. I have achieved the following series of scientific research results. The following monographs have been published.

Three monographs in Chinese version were published and distributed in the domestic nation

Thirteen monographs in English version were published and distributed in the international.

These 16 monographs are our hard journey, hard climbing, step by step, four different scientific research stages, four different levels of mountain results.

1. Xu Ze etc (the first monograph published in the 67-year-old flower year) *"New understanding and new model of cancer treatment"* Hubei Science and Technology Press, January 2001

2. Xu Ze etc (the second monograph published in the 73-year-old ancient rare year) *"New concept and new method of cancer metastasis treatment"* published by Beijing People's Military Medical Press, January 2006; "Three One hundred original book certificate" was issued by the People's Republic of China Publishing House in April 2007

3. Xu Ze etc (the third book published in the 78-year-old ancient year) *"New concept and new method of cancer treatment"* published by Beijing People's Military Medical Press, October 2011; later the American medical doctor Dr. Bin Wu translated into English, the English edition was published in Washington, DC on March 26, 2013.

4. Xu Ze etc (the third edition of the special edition of the English version was published in the 80-year-old year) *"New Concept and New Way Of Treatment of Cancer"*, published in USA in March 2013 in English, internationally distributed

5. Xu Ze etc (the fifth book published at the age of 82) **"On Innovation of Treatment of Cancer"**, published in USA in December 2015, full English version, global distribution

6. Xu Ze etc (published the sixth monograph at the age of 83) **"New Concept and New Way of Treatment of Cancer Metastais"** published on August 2016 in USA in English, global issued

7. Xu Ze etc (the seventh book was published at the age of 83) **"The Road To Over Come Cancer"**, published in USA in December 2016 in English, published worldwide.

8. Xu Ze etc (published the eighth monograph at the age of 86) **"Condense Wisdom and Conquer Cancer for the Benefit of Mankind"**

Volume I: How to overcome cancer? How to prevent cancer? In December 2017
Volume II: How to overcome cancer? How to treat cancer? In February 2018
} *Published in USA in English and distributed globly*

9. Xu Ze etc (the ninth monograph was published in the year of 87) **"The New progress in Cancer Treatment"**, published in USA in June 2018 in English, globally distributed

10. Xu Ze etc (the eleventh monograph was published in the year of 87 years old) **"Conquer Cancer and Launch The Total attack to Cancer"** in USA in November 2018 Published, full English, global distribution(Volume I)

11. Xu Ze etc(the twelfth monograph was published in the year of 88 years old) **"Walked Out of the New Road to Conquer Cancer" (part I)** (Volume II) in USA in January 2019 published, full English, global distribution

Walked Out of the New Way of Cancer Treatment with Immune Regulation and Control of Combination of Chinese and Western Medicine

12. Xu Ze etc(the thirteenth monograph was published in the year of 88 years old) **Walked Out of the New Road to Conquer Cancer(part II)(Volume III)** in USA in January 2019 published, full English, global distribution
Walked Out of the New Way of Cancer Treatment with Immune Regulation and Control of the Combination of Chinese and Western Medicine

13. Xu Ze etc(the fourteenth monograph was published in the year of 88 years old) **The Research on Anticancer Traditional Chinese Medication with Immune Regulation and Control** (Volume IV) in USA in February 2019 published, full English, global distribution ——Experimental Research and Clinical Application Verification

14. Xu Ze etc(the fifteenth monograph was published in the year of 88 years old) **Innovation on Clinical Application Theory of Cancer Prevention and Treatment Research in the 21st Century** (Volume V) in USA in February 2019 published, full English, global distribution

15. Xu Ze etc(the sixteenth monograph was published in the year of 88 years old) *Build up the multidisciplinary and the science city of the research base with related to cancer research for conquering cancer* in USA in March 2019 published, full English, global distribution

ACKNOWLEDGEMENTS

This book is for all of people who concern human being health. We are deeply grateful to all of people who like our new ways to improve our human being health.

I appreciated all of the people who encourage us to finish all of these books. My life is extremely difficult years and years even if I work very hard, *for example, I live in USA and I have to look for XXXX all the time and I don't have stable income and in the evening in Winter it was extremely cold of sticking into my bone in my room while these book were finished. Many times I woke up by this cold. Thank everyone who helps me and encourage me to work hard to help others. I face the disasters in my life, however I still work hard.*

I pray and pray for God's support. Challenges! I am a brave solider to prevent others. I love my daughter Lily Xu and always give the concise idea and I learn from her such as she loves challenges and she loves to think in detail and she has wisdoms and loves to read and learns things logically, etc.

My daughter **Lily Xu** gave me many smart and creative ideas while we were finishing this book and she is really bright light for my life and gives me encouragement such as during the cold weather she came to all of the dance and music and other classes after the regular school and during the weekend to get extra study. Lily Xu drew all of the pictures such as the Thymus and cancer stages and cancer metastasis steps and stages etc. **The characteristics of she loves the challenge** and **her judgment always encourages me to continue working hard to move on**.

I would like to express our sincere gratitude to the following:

1. All of Authorhouse staffs
2. All of the persons who encourage me.

Bin Wu, M.D., Ph.D

05-24-2019 in Baltimore, Maryland in USA

FOREWORD

- This series of monographs is not written in pens, but it is made with hard work.

- In these monographs all of contents come from clinical practice experience and lessons, review, reflect, and practice real knowledge.

- In these monographs all of the contents come from the experimental research results of our own laboratory and the experiment produces the achievement and the results.

- In these monographs, all of the contents are the true record of scientific research thinking and scientific practice from experiment to clinical, and then from clinical to experimental research thinking and scientific practice, and it is the summary of experimental research and clinical validation data, then it is rising to the theoretical essence, proposing new discoveries, new understandings, new theories, which these clinical practical innovation theories can be used to guide clinical treatment. All should be transferred to clinical applications through transformation medicine or translational medicine to guide clinical treatment work and benefit patients.

- In these monographs all of the contents are the summary and collation of my own treatment practice experience in more than half a century and many years of experimental research data, then made into the collection of books and became into the different volumes. The scientific research results and the scientific and technological innovation series are my own materials, some of which are international initiatives, original innovation. Some are internationally advanced, independent innovation, and have independent intellectual property rights.

- In these monographs all of the contents are fully compliant with transform or translational medicine content.

Our 60-year scientific research route is from clinical → experimental → clinical → re-experiment → re-clinical, back to clinical to solve clinical practical problems, our research model is fully in line with this new medical research model.

Translational medicine or transform medicine:

Translational medicine has developed rapidly in the world in recent years. This new medical research model advocates patient-centered, discovers and raises questions from clinical work, conducts in-depth basic research, and *then quickly shifts basic research results to clinical applications to improve overall medical care and ultimately benefit patients.*

In the ministry of Health the Former Minister Chen Yu has analyzed the connotation of translational medicine:

First of all, translational medicine is a science that explores the mechanisms of disease occurrence, development, and health protection promotion **through laboratory-to-clinical and clinical-to-laboratory two-way channels** *to explore new prevention strategies*.

Secondly, it is necessary to transform scientific research results into the practical intervention means, techniques, and programs that *can be used for clinical or public health, so that they can be popularized*.

The World Health Organization proposes that medicine in the 21st century should not continue to focus on diseases, but should be human health as the main research direction. Academician Chen Yu pointed out: **the transformation of the health service model should shift from the treatment of the late stage of the major illness** *into being the prevention as the main pions*, **and move the gate or checkpoint barrier forward and sink the center of gravity. Strengthening preventive medical research is a major issue of the transformation of the medical model in China and in the globe as well.**

The focus of translational medicine research in China is that the modernization and internationalization of traditional Chinese medicine and traditional Chinese medicine is one of the key contents of translational medicine research in China.

Xu Ze

April 2019 in China • Hubei • Wuhan

XZ-C proposed that in order to conquer cancer and to launch the total attack It is necessary to establish cancer prevention research institute and carry out cancer prevention system engineering, which is the first time to be proposed in the world.

It should conduct cancer prevention research, find cancer-causing factors, and detect the source of carcinogens or carcinogenic factors. And it should try to stop the damage caused by these carcinogenic factors. The Cancer Research Institute should conduct cancer prevention research, and there is a lot of content that is urgently needed to be studied.

It should track the source of carcinogens or carcinogenic factors.

In the process of searching the cause of cancer and the occurrence of conditions of cancer, *the most prominent thing is that it was found that more than 90% of cancers are caused by environmental factors.*

1. Relationship between air pollution and cancer

Humans have developed tens of millions of tons of coal, oil and natural gas as fuel and energy. In the process of production and living life such as thermal power generation, smelting steel, automobiles, aircraft and other means of transportation and family life fuel, etc. **A large amount of tar, bituminous coal, dust and other harmful substances are discharged into the atmosphere around the clock, causing air pollution.**

Air pollution can cause many diseases, especially respiratory track diseases, the most serious is lung cancer.

2. Water pollution and cancer

The pollution of water quality is mainly caused by industrial and agricultural production and urban sewage. There are many types of pollutants in the water. **Pesticides and pesticides are one of the important pollutants in water bodies. Surfactants in neutral detergents also have a cancer-promoting effect.**

3. Soil pollution and cancer

A large amount of industrial waste water residue and pesticides and fertilizers are injected into the soil, **which deteriorates soil quality, accumulates poisons, and poses a threat to human health. It is also a carcinogenic factor.**

4. Chemistry and cancer

5. Physical factors and cancer

6. Biological factors and cancer

7. Diet and cancer

8. Lifestyle and cancer

9. Clothing, food, housing, travel, house decoration, etc. and cancer

The effective way in which so many carcinogens or carcinogenic factors should be studied.

It should study these sources of pollution and try to stop at the source.

It should study these carcinogenic mechanisms and their carcinogenic effects.

It should study the preventive methods of how to reduce or prevent these carcinogens.

Conquer cancer   Launch the total attack

<< The Science City ---- Multidisciplinary and Research base with the Cancer Research Group for conquering cancer and Launching the total attack of Cancer>>

Total Design • Blueprint • Preparation Work
(One)

XZ-C proposes:

In order to conquer cancer, it is necessary to create the research institute of the environmental protection cancer and to carry out cancer prevention system engineering.

First

how to prevent cancer, I see one

How to conquer cancer and how to prevent cancer by I see
How to prevent cancer? What to prevent? How to prevent it?

Professor Xu Ze proposed how to overcome cancer, how to prevent cancer by I see: (1 - 3)

(1) Situation analysis 1

The incidence of cancer is rising

How to overcome cancer? How to prevent cancer by I see one:

How to prevent cancer? The incidence of cancer is rising.

1. From what I have seen in my 85-year-old society this year:

I deeply felt that the incidence of cancers that are currently threatening people's health is on the rise, or the incidence of cancer, a major disease that threatens people's health, is rising.

(1) I came to Zhongnan Tongji Medical College in Wuhan in 1951. I graduated from Tongji Medical College in 1956 and was assigned to the surgical work of the Affiliated Hospital of Hubei College of Traditional Chinese Medicine. I has successively served as director of surgery, professor, and director of the Institute of Experimental Surgery of Hubei College of Traditional Chinese Medicine.

When the Central South Tongji Medical College moved from Shanghai to Wuhan in 1951, at that time, for the teaching, in order to find a case of lung cancer to train students, it was difficult to find one case even if the phone call was made to the hospital one week earlier.

At that time (from the 1950s to the 1960s), all hospitals in Wuhan had no oncology department and no oncologists. Only one hospital in Wuhan had a medical doctor to see blood diseases. There is a gynecologist in Tongji Hospital and also look at gynecological tumors.

But now, (65 years later) cancer is a common disease, frequently-occurring disease, more common in each hospital, cancer patients are all queued for registration, and all the top three hospitals have oncology departments busy with cancer treatment. I have been doing tumor surgery for 60 years. The more patients are treated, the more patients come. Our physicians should think hard and review reflections. Why is this? Why are patients getting more and more? What is the reason? Or what factors lead to an increase in morbidity? What should I do?

I have been in medical clinical work for 60 years. It has been 30 years of experimental basic research and clinical verification to overcome cancer. I have deeply realized that cancer should not only pay attention to treatment, *__but also should pay attention to prevention, in order to stop at the source, in order to promote the decline of cancer incidence.__*

The way out for cancer treatment is "three early" (early detection, early diagnosis, early treatment), and the way out to conquer cancer is prevention.

(2) Situation analysis 2

The incidence of cancer is related to the environment.

__How to overcome cancer How to prevent cancer by I see two:__

Cancer incidence is related to the environment.

Then, how should we prevent it? What to prevent? How to prevent it? Where is the target or "target" of cancer prevention? How to control? What to control? How to control? Where is the target or "target" of cancer control?

It must have specific cancer prevention targets, clear goals, and operability. The motivation must be consistent with the effect.

Currently the more patients are treated, the more patients will occur. The incidence is rising, 90% of this is related to the environment. Why is that? Professor Xu's goal or "target" for cancer prevention should aim research and discuss the carcinogenic factors (external environment, internal environment) of the environment.

1. <u>Why does the increase in cancer incidence have a relationship with the environment?</u>

<u>Because cancer is a malignant change of abnormal cells, it is caused by external factors (external environment) or internal factors (internal environment).</u> Cells are always in a controlled dynamic balance of proliferation, survival, and death during normal development. **However, under the influence of external factors (external environment) or internal factors (internal environment), the proliferation of a cell is abnormal, breaking through the normal restriction mechanism and rapidly proliferating, forming a tissue mass, which is formed by abnormal proliferation. The group is called a tumor.** Tumors have benign and malignant, and only proliferate without spreading, called benign tumors; but not only abnormally rapid proliferation, but also cells can spread and metastasize, called malignant tumors, malignant tumors are cancer.

2. The cause of cancer is related to the carcinogenic factors of the external environment and the internal environment.

After years of worldwide research, people have now achieved a consensus:

That is, carcinogenesis is an evolution process of multi-factor, multi-stage and multi-gene which is the external as one side and the body genetic (substance) as one side.

<u>The so-called external factors refer to factors other than the cytogenetic factors themselves, including chemical factors, physical factors, biological (bacterial, viral, etc.) factors in the living environment other than the human body, as well as human lifestyles and eating habits, as well as physical Internal environment, such as hormonal status, disease infection, and mental factors.</u>

Genetics refers to the genetic material DNA or genes, which leads to two basic factors in the development of cancer:

One is an intrinsic genetic factor; the other is an external environmental factor. Most cancers are the result of a combination of these two factors.

3. **If we have a deeper understanding of the causes of cancer, then we can come up with more valuable suggestions in the future:**

<u>It should be how to prevent what or which the carcinogenic factors are, how to monitor what the carcinogenic factors are, even how to clear what the carcinogenic factors are so as to keep us away from cancer and prevent cancer,</u> such as it should not smoke, it should not eat pickles and smoked products and strong sun exposure should be avoided. All of these are an important way to reduce the incidence of cancer in the future.

The Analysis from the above situation (1)

It is suggested or prompted as the following:

1. In Wuhan City in the 1950s and 1960s, there were few cancer patients, neither oncology nor oncologists.

But now (65 years later) cancer is a common disease, frequently-occurring disease, patients are queued for registration, each of the top three hospitals have oncology, all of which are busy with cancer treatment.

It is proofed that : The incidence of cancer is rising.

2. It should analyze that what the reason of the cancer incidence to rise is? what the cause is or what causes the cancer incidence to rise? or what factors lead to an increase in cancer incidence?

Why is it? what should it be done? **Whether can the factors that contribute to the rise in cancer incidence be found through In-depth analysis from this point or not, so that it is to find a way to prevent cancer and control cancer?**

The analysis from the above situation (2)

It is suggested or prompted as the following:

1. **Cancer is a malignant change of abnormal proliferation of cells, which is caused by external factors (external environment) or internal factors (internal environment).**

The so-called external factors refer to factors other than the cytogenetic factors themselves, including:

chemical factors, physical factors, biological (bacteria, viruses) and other factors in the living environment other than the human body, as well as people's lifestyles, eating habits, and the internal environment of the body such as endocrine hormones, mental factors and so on.

2. To analyze what the cause of the cancer incidence is rising? or what causes the cancer incidence to rise?

Nowadays people's living standards are constantly improving, and various high-tech products have brought us a better life. At the same time, they have brought about a large number of chemical, physical and biological environmental carcinogens. Various carcinogens enter the human body or various carcinogenic factors affect the human body. People seem to be shrouded in the oceans of environmentally harmful carcinogens.

From this point of view, the rise in the incidence of cancer is causey or there are reasons to be found that the incidence of cancer is rising. The target or "target" of cancer prevention is also very clear, very specific, how should cancer be prevented? How to control? What to prevent? It is clear, specific, and operable.

It's just that when some people talk about cancer, and they seem to be arrogant; others are insensitive and do what they do in life.

Cancer is not terrible. What is terrible is that we don't have a simple basic knowledge of cancer prevention, because most cancers are preventable.

(3) Analysis of the situation 3

It should improve external factors (external environment) and internal factors (internal environment) to prevention of carcinogenic factors

How to conquer cancer and how to prevent cancer by I see three:

(3) - Prevention should be carried out from the improvement of external factors (external environment) and internal factors (internal environment).

How to prevent? We should prevent carcinogenic factors from the above external factors (external environment) and internal factors (internal environment).

Professor Xu Ze proposed the establishment of an innovative cancer prevention research institute and an innovative cancer prevention system project. This is an unprecedented work and must be practiced in person to seek health and welfare for mankind.

How to implement the creation of this cancer research institute?

Professor Xu Ze XZ-C proposed the general design of cancer prevention and proposed cancer prevention system engineering:

(1) Personal prevention:

It should be to improve cancer prevention knowledge (see separate article).

(2) The government should carry out cancer prevention engineering

1 What is cancer prevention project?

a. That is, the above-mentioned departments will monitor, characterize, quantify, and set the bottom line standards for the causative cancer factors, and prevent them or stop it, even legislating, to legislate, and each division of labor is responsible.

b. This requires that the government is in charge of it and the government arranges the engineering details of the cancer prevention system.

c. Each department is divided for the labor and work for being responsible for. The Cancer Research Institute conducts technical monitoring.

d. Macro, micro, ultra-micro, sampling, providing effective reporting.

2. From which departments and scopes are they detected?

Xu Ze proposed that it should be tested whether there are carcinogenic factors from clothing, food, housing, and transportation.

a. [clothing]:

- Light industry department is responsible for receiving investigations and tests:

It is to detect the causing Ca factors such as clothing, cosmetics, toys, etc. If it is exceeding the standard levels, it should be warned or stopped.

b. [Food]:

- The agricultural department and the food department are responsible for receiving investigation and research and it is to detect water, soil, fertilizer, agricultural genetic modification, food, fish, meat, chicken, duck, packaged food, food, oil, feed materials... carcinogenic factors.

c. [Residence]:

- The building construction department is responsible for receiving investigations and tests:

monitoring of carcinogenic factors such as decoration materials, supplies, and design, and those who exceed the standard will be warned and blocked.

d. [Travel]:

- The industrial department is responsible for receiving investigations for trains, automobiles, aircrafts, ... tail gas hazards. It should not be allowed to exceed the standard through detection and it should be legislated.

e. Environment:

The environmental protection department shall be responsible for, support, receive for being monitored and investigated the pollution such as garbage disposal, air pollution, water pollution, factory chimneys, etc. by the cancer prevention research institute. It should be from macroscopic and microscopic to monitor and to qualitatively and quantitatively detect carcinogen content. Those which are exceeding the standard should be warned or blocked.

f. Education department:

University, middle school and elementary school teachers should be models as teachers

No smoking allowed
(Smoking has a lot of harm and no benefit,
Smoking is an unknowledgable performance,
Smoking harms others and harms people)

University, middle school and elementary students

The content of the textbook is plus:

> physical hygiene
> Health care, basic moral knowledge
> Cancer prevention and anti-cancer and other knowledge

g. **Professor Xu Ze proposed that research ethics should be advocated, medicine is benevolence, and ethics is the first**

Research ethics:

Products should have ethical standards

Standard:

It should be based on the standard of not damaging human health

Basic ethics:

All products are harmless to people and do not harm people's health, especially for children.

(To be beautiful and having bird and flowery living environment and surviving environment)

h. **the health administrative department protects lives and protects health, and it should lead, dominant, support, guide cancer prevention measures, cancer**

prevention engineering, cancer prevention detection, cancer prevention monitoring, cancer is a human disaster, people all over the world are eager to one day to overcome cancer. It is urgent to hope that experts and scholars can find out cancer prevention measures to keep people away from cancer.

Cancer is a disaster for all mankind. It must fight globally. The people of the world must work together. **Human beings should not sit still. Physicians should not do nothing. The health administrative department should not do nothing. It should lead and guide the series of cancer prevention research projects, and moving forward together, work together, c**omplementary advantages, lead and guide the fight against cancer, launch the general attack.

Environmental pollution, air pollution, water pollution, and the incidence of cancer are rising. This is not a country or a region. It is a global problem. This is a by-product and episode in industrial development. It should be analyzed and researched. The World Health Organization should be invited to lead research a project to prevent all environmental pollution from causing cancer, and to defend the beautiful living environment on which human beings depend for survival, and the harmonious and friendly environment in which human beings depend for survival, and to stay away from cancer.

(4) Situation Analysis 4

Establishing the Environmental and Cancer Research Group

How to overcome cancer how to prevent cancer? I see four:

It should sep up the Environmental and Cancer Research Group.

How to implement the establishment of the Cancer Prevention Research Institute?

The Environmental and Cancer Research Group should be established:

(1) It is to investigate and test common cancer risk factors and to conduct an intensive intervention study.

(2) **It is to monitor pollution-causing cancer data and to research and develop cancer prevention and cancer control measures.**

Aim For:

a, food, the eaten things, packaging, additives

b, water pollution, beverages

c, house decoration, materials

d, air pollution, factory chimneys, car tail steam

e, soil, fertilizer, genetic modification

(3) Monitoring environmental pollution carcinogenic data and researching cancer prevention measures and R&D intervention(researching and developing intervention)

(4) Establishing a cancer prevention and cancer control information and communication report (publication) - "Cancer Prevention Mass Medicine"

Preventing cancer from the big living environment and the small living environment, and staying away from cancer.

(5) Several tasks:

a, monitoring environmental pollution caused by cancer (data)

b, spot check cancer incidence rate in high cancer area

c, founding cancer prevention and anti-cancer information newsletter

d, To research and to develop cancer prevention technology, tools, products

e, science (cancer prevention) publicity and education

f, "three early" popular learning

g, how to self-early discovery

(6) Several aspects:

a, from clothing, food, shelter, anti-cancer

b, from the big environment of life to prevent cancer

c, from the small living environment to prevent cancer

d, from life behavior, life hobbies, living habits to prevent cancer

(7) Three key points in the 21st century cancer prevention:

a, smoking ban (smoking cessation) - "smoking has thousands of harm and no benefits"

b, limited alcohol - limit the amount of alcohol

c, weight loss - not suitable for obesity

(5) Situation analysis 5

Relationship between environment and cancer

How to implement the creation of cancer prevention system project for cancer prevention research?

First, we must understand the history record of the relationship between environmental pollution and cancer.

Xu Ze proposed in Chapter 38 of his third book<< New Essentials and New Methods in Cancer Therapy>>:

The situation analysis:

---------the relationship between environment and cancer

In the process of searching for the cancer cause and the condition of the occurrence and development of cancer, human beings have carried out extensive exploration and accumulated rich knowledge. It was found that more than 90% of cancers are caused by or closely related to environmental factors.

The environment in which humans live includes the natural environment and the social environment. The natural environment, that is, the various natural factors surrounding people, such as everyone breathing air, drinking water and food, these common physical environment is called the big environment. Everyone must engage in certain work and adopt a certain lifestyle, such as occupation, living habits and hobbies, to form a living environment called a small environment. Whether it is a large environment or a small environment, it is the external environment on which human beings depend for survival and activity. The physiological condition of the human body is called the internal environment. The external environment substances have a close relationship with the internal environment through the uptake, digestion, absorption, metabolism and excretion of the organism, which has a huge impact on the human body. The external environment substances have a close relationship with the internal environment through the ingestion, digestion, absorption, metabolism and excretion of the organism, which has a huge impact on the human body.

There are many examples of how to prove the relationship between environmental pollution and cancer.

In 1775, Dr. Pott of the United Kingdom confirmed that there were many cases of scrotal skin cancer among workers who cleaned the chimney, mainly due to long-term exposure to coal tar. This is the first historical example of linking cancer to environmental factors.

After 100 years, German doctor Volkltlayl also realized that the high incidence of skin cancer among workers may be related to exposure to coal tar.

In 1907, some scholars discovered that sun exposure was associated with skin cancer, and first reported epidemiological studies of sunlight and skin cancer. The researchers observed early on that the crew were exposed to solar radiation and caused chronic skin disease. This is a very common phenomenon, and it has been later confirmed by animal models that sunlight and ultraviolet rays can cause skin cancer.

In 1915, an animal model of the first chemical-induced tumor was established. Repeated application of tar can cause skin cancer in rabbits.

This study added experimental evidence for the establishment of a chemical carcinogenic doctrine based on the scrotal cancer in chimney cleaners in 1775.

Later, the active ingredient, coal tar, was confirmed and isolated.

In the 20th century, it was confirmed that high-initiated bladder cancer was produced among workers producing Methylnaphthylamine, ethyl naphthylamine and benzidine dyes, and <u>almost all workers who had engaged in such occupations subsequently developed bladder cancer</u>.

In 1930, the first chemical carcinogen, benzopyrene, was separated from coal tar. Known carcinogenic environmental substances, coal tar, are separated into different components, and the carcinogenic effects of these chemical components are clarified by animal model experiments.

In 1938, the study found that the chemical carcinogenesis process was divided into two different stages, that is, the excitation or initiate phase and the promotion phase, non-specific stimulator promotes the occurrence of tumors after excitation by low dose of carcinogen, for example, tar or papillomavirus is applied to the ears of rabbits.

In 1940, researchers found that limiting calories can reduce the incidence of murine or mouse tumors. It was proved that the intake of calories can cause the development of several tumors, such as breast cancer, liver cancer, and skin cancer induced by benzopyrene. Until today's obesity is prevalent in the world, this work has once again received the attention of people.

In 1950, epidemiological studies found that smoking was associated with lung cancer. Retrospective analysis of lung cancer patients with smoking habits has shown that smoking is associated with lung cancer.

Later studies in male doctors showed that smoking has a significant relationship with lung cancer mortality. Smoking has now proven to be a risk factor for many cancers, increasing cancer mortality by around 30%.

In 1958, <u>food additives</u> banned by food additive improvement agencies were shown to induce cancer in humans or animals.

In 1964, American surgeon Luther L Terry suggested that smoking is associated with lung cancer.

<u>Vinyl chloride is the main raw material for the plastics industry</u>. It was not until 1974 that scientists discovered that **<u>this chemical was a potentially strong carcinogen that caused liver cancer</u>**.

Epidemiological investigations in recent decades have found that many occupational workers are exposed to carcinogens in the production environment, and the incidence of cancer in some areas is greatly increased. When these occupational exposures are eliminated or avoided, the onset of these cancers can be gradually reduced or even disappeared, indicating that environmental factors play a major role in tumorigenesis.

The long-term effects of various environmental factors other than the human body are the main causes of most cancers. Therefore, the effects of these environmental, living and behavioral factors on the human body should be minimized and away from cancer.

Let's talk about the serious impact of environmental pollution such as air pollution, water pollution and soil pollution on human carcinogenesis.

1). Air pollution and cancer in environmental pollution:

Human beings can't live without air every minute and every second of their lives or human life is inseparable from air every minute and every second. Air pollution can cause many diseases, especially respiratory diseases, including the most severe lung cancer.

At the beginning of the 20th century, lung cancer mainly occurred in a few occupational environments for mining and smelting. After the First World War, lung cancer mortality began to rise. In the late 1930s or entering the late 1930s, **with the development of modern industry, atmospheric pollution, occupational carcinogens, tobacco and cigarette production or consumption are soaring, male patients in western industrialized countries experience a rapid increase in lung cancer mortality or have rapidly increased their mortality due to lung cancer.** In England the patient's lung cancer mortality rate was 10/10 million in 1930, 53/100,000 in 1950, 99.7/100,000 in 1966, and 120.3/100,000 in 1975. It has grown 12 times in the 45 years from 1930 to 1975.

From 1934 to 1974, American male lung cancer jumped from the fifth death cause to the top. The mortality rate increased from 3.0/100,000 to 54.5/10, an increase of 17 times; female lung cancer moved from the 8th to the top 3, and the mortality rate increased from 2/100,000 to 12.4/100,000, an increase of 5.2 times.

By the early 1980s, lung cancer in 24 countries and regions such as the United Kingdom, France, the Netherlands, Germany and North America is listed as the leading cause of death in patients with malignant tumors.

Since the middle of the 20th century, it has been a rapid upward trend led by the high incidence of lung cancer in western industrialized countries.

In industrialized countries, harmful gases such as power generation, steelmaking, automobiles, aircraft, fuel, energy, and large amounts of smoke <u>are emitted into the atmosphere, polluting the air, and people are irritated by the respiratory tract, leading to an increase in the incidence and mortality of lung cancer</u>.

2). water pollution in environmental pollution and cancer:

Humans are inseparable from water every moment in production activities and life. The pollution of water quality is mainly caused by industrial and agricultural production and urban sewage. In China, industrial pollution has intensified due to the rapid development of township and village enterprises.

According to the survey, many key rivers are increasingly polluted. **Fertilizers, pesticides and pesticides in agricultural production cause serious pollution of water quality.**

Some rural areas in China have the habit of using pond water. **A study <u>in Qidong County, Jiangsu Province, found that high incidence of liver cancer in this area is related to drinking pond water</u>. Similar reports have been made in Fusui County, Guangxi. <u>This shows that water pollution is associated with high incidence of liver cancer</u>. Haining City, Zhejiang Province also found that the risk of colon cancer in drinking pond water was more than 7 times higher than that of drinking well water.**

In recent years, due to advances in water quality analysis technology, **<u>it has been found that more than 100 kinds of organic substances in water are carcinogenic, cancer-promoting and mutagenic.</u>** It has been confirmed in animal experiments that the following compounds can be added to drinking water to cause liver cancer, such as **666 or hexachlorocyclohexane, carbon tetrachloride, chloroform, trichloroethylene, tetrachloroethylene, trichloroethane, and the like.**

In addition, some freshwater algae toxins, **<u>such as blue-green algae, have been found to have a significant effect on liver cancer</u>**.

The Sangde fish pond area in Shunde, Foshan, Guangdong, is low-lying.

It is easy to accumulate water, <u>water quality pollution is more serious. The incidence of liver cancer in residents is high.</u> The neighboring Siping residents drink deep well water, the water quality is good, and the incidence of liver cancer is relatively low. According to a large number of research data from the World Health Organization and the International Association for Research on Cancer, drinking substandard water can induce or promote cancer. Tests have shown that drinking water contains more nickel, which is more susceptible to oral cancer, throat cancer and colorectal cancer; the drinking water containing a large amount of cadmium is susceptible to esophageal cancer, laryngeal cancer, lung cancer; the water including many lead-containing chemical elements are prone to stomach cancer, intestinal or colon cancer, ovarian cancer and various lymphomas; the one containing more iron and zinc chemical elements is susceptible to esophageal cancer.

3). Environmental chemical pollution and cancer - chemical carcinogen:

A chemical carcinogen refers to a chemical substance that induces tumor formation.

The chemical carcinogen problem in the middle of the 20th century has caused widespread concern. The problem of chemical carcinogenesis in the middle of the 20th century has caused widespread concern, mainly because of the increasing incidence of morbidity and mortality in modern times, the age of cancer, and the discovery that environmental chemical pollution is closely related to the incidence of cancer. **The World Health Organization also pointed out that 80% to 90% of human cancers are related to environmental factors, mainly chemical factors.**

The following are chemical substances that have been researched and proven to be carcinogenic.

Vinyl chloride:

In 1974, people began to realize that this substance is the cause of occupational cancer. The Experimental Study shows that among the experimental animals exposed to vinyl chloride, cancers of liver cancer, brain cancer, kidney cancer, lung cancer, and lymphatic system were found. However, the personnel concerned failed to recognize the hazards of these substances in time from these important experimental results, and thus failed to take timely measures to protect workers.

Until recently, the ban on the use of vinyl chloride sprays and plastic factories has also changed the production process to prevent workers from being exposed.

In here, it should be pointed out here that vinyl chloride is an important raw material for records, packaging materials, medical test tubes, household appliances, bathroom equipment and many other plastic products. Plastic products are not inherently dangerous, **but workers in vinyl chloride plants are 200 times more likely to have liver cancer than the average person.**

Benzene:

This is a harmful chemical that destroys the hematopoietic function of the bone marrow. Aplastic anemia can occur in repeated exposure to benzene. This disease can become leukemia after a long time. In 1928, the first case of "benzene leukemia" was discovered.

Other countries have also shown that benzene is an occupational hazard. Italian scientists reported 200 years ago that **the risk of leukemia in printing and shoe factories is 20 times higher than in the general population.**

Certain activities and certain hobbies in human daily life are often closely related to environmental carcinogen polycyclic aromatic hydrocarbons. The production of polycyclic aromatic hydrocarbons by smoking is an important factor in inducing human lung cancer. In the cooking process of frying, burning, and smoking of fat and oil foods,

there are also carcinogenic polycyclic aromatic hydrocarbons, which are carcinogens that pose a great threat to human health. We must pay enough attention to them.

In addition, **benzopyrene in asphalt and hot asphalt is associated to the high incidence of cancer in the road workers and roof workers and waterproofing worker. Agricultural workers are exposed to a variety of pesticides, herbicides and fertilizers, some are known to be human carcinogens,** some have been induced in experimental animals, and others have been shown to be mutagens after short-term trials. Pesticides enter the food chain and accumulate in biological systems.

4). Physical factors in environmental pollution and cancer - ionizing radiation:

With the development of science and technology, the frequent tests of nuclear tests, the application of nuclear energy and radionuclides are increasing, and the amount of radioactive substances entering the human environment is also increasing. Therefore, the environmental pollution caused by ionizing radiation has received more and more attention.

The so-called ionizing radiation refers to certain radioactive materials that emit radiation during the metamorphosis process. This kind of ray energy can provide the sufficient amount of energy for the atoms and molecules in the absorbing substance are ionized. Some ionizing radiation is electromagnetic radiation, such as X-rays and gamma(γ) rays.

The nuclear tests with the artificial radiation sources have that increase environmental radioactive contamination; nuclear fuel is mined, processed and reprocessed, such as ore mining, with radon and radioactive dust polluting the atmosphere. Due to energy shortages in nuclear power plants, more and more countries are developing nuclear power plants. This nuclear power industry has radioactive waste gas, waste water and waste slag, which will pollute the environment if not handled properly.

Radionuclides are widely used in industry, agriculture, and medicine, and the resulting radioactive waste can also pollute the environment.

The effects of ionizing radiation on the human body are mainly physical injuries such as chronic radiation sickness, malignant tumors, cataracts, and decreased fertility. Radiation is carcinogenic, and its carcinogenic effect has a long incubation period, such as leukemia, skin cancer, lung cancer, and bone cancer. Genetic damage causes hereditary diseases in the offspring.

5). Carcinogens that enter food from environmental pollution:

With the development of science and technology, the food processing process is increasingly industrialized, and the external environment or the manufacturing process itself may cause various foreign substances, including chemical and biological carcinogens, to contaminate food.

In the processing of food raw materials, artificial additives are added, and smoking, frying, baking, etc. are used, and as a result, carcinogenic hybrids may appear in the food.

Food products are often stored and transported to reach consumers, thus providing an additional source of carcinogen-contaminated food.

Studying the sources of carcinogens on human food and how to eliminate such pollution is a very important issue.

(6) Situation analysis 6

What are the carcinogenic factors in the environment? How to prevent it?

How to prevent? What is an important part of cancer prevention?

As early as the 1980s, many experts and scholars at home and abroad believed *that more than 90% of cancers were caused by environmental factors. Protecting and restoring a good environment is an important part of preventing cancer.*

How to prevent cancer? How to prevent it?

It must first understand what the carcinogenic factors are and its carcinogenic process so that it can only propose preventive measures.

1. **Chemical factors are the main cause of human cancer, and 90% of human cancers are caused by environmental factors. More than 75% of them are chemical factors.**

The earliest observations of chemical factors and human cancers can be traced back to the 1870s. Percivall Port found that men who had been chimney sweepers in childhood had an increased rate of scrotal cancer. Although the nature of carcinogens was not known at the time, this finding by Port suggests a link between occupational exposure and tumor onset. Since then, many examples have clarified the relationship between various chemical carcinogens and human tumors, providing a series of experimental evidence for scientists to study and understand chemical carcinogenesis.

2. **What is a chemical carcinogen?**

It refers to a chemical substance that has the ability to induce cancer formation.

The chemical carcinogenic problem in the middle of the 20th century has caused widespread concern, and it has been found that environmental chemical pollution is closely related to the incidence of cancer.

The World Health Organization also pointed out that 90% of human cancers are related to environmental factors, mainly chemical factors. For treating the diseases, it is advisable to understand the cause of the disease. Anti-cancer is

also the first to understand what the carcinogenic factors in the environment are, how to avoid?

Common chemical carcinogens mainly involve the following 11 types of chemicals(types and sample of chemical carcinogens):

1), alkylating agent

Mustard gas, chloromethyl ether, formaldehyde, ethylene oxide, diethyl sulfate, ethylene, benzene, butadiene, carcinogenic alkylating agents

2), Polycyclic aromatic hydrocarbons

Benzopyrene, dimethyl benzoquinone, diphenyl hydrazine, 3-methyl cholesteric, etc. and coal tar pitch

3), Aromatic amines

Benzidine, ethyl naphthylamine, nitrobiphenyl

4), metal and metalloid

Arsenic, nickel, chromium, antimony, cadmium, selenium

5), mold and plant toxins

Aflatoxin, microcystins, etc.

6), nitrosamines and nitrosamides

7), asbestos and silica

8), hobby goods

Cigarettes, tobacco, betel nuts, excess alcohol and beverages

9), food pyrolysis products

10), drugs

Including certain hormones

11), cancer-promoting substances

Some chemicals have only a cancer-promoting effect and should be classified as such, such as croton oil and its purified phorbol ester. Some cancer-promoting substances also have a priming effect.

3. There are many kinds of chemical carcinogens.

In order to systematically and deeply study chemical carcinogens, it is necessary to classify them. There are mainly three classification methods, which are based on the action mode of chemical carcinogens, the relationship between chemical carcinogens and human tumors, and chemical classification.

(1) Classification by the action mode of chemical carcinogens

According to the action mode of chemical carcinogens, they can be divided into direct carcinogens, indirect carcinogens and carcinogens.

1) direct carcinogen

It refers to a chemical carcinogen that can directly affect the cells of the body after it enters the body and can directly affect the cells in the body. These chemical carcinogens have strong carcinogenicity and rapid oncogenic effects, and are often used for malignant transformation studies of cells in vitro such as various carcinogenic alkylating agents, nitrosamide carcinogens and the like.

2) indirect carcinogens

It refers to the chemical carcinogen that is activated by the in vivo microsomal mixed function oxidase after it enters the human body and becomes a chemically active form with carcinogenic effects such as chemical carcinogens are widely present in the external environment, and are commonly found to be carcinogenic polycyclic aromatic hydrocarbons, aromatic amines, nitrosamines, and the like.

3) tumor promoters, also known as tumor promoters

The carcinogen alone acts on the body without carcinogenic effects, but can promote other carcinogens to induce tumor formation. Common promotional items are croton oil (phorbol diester), saccharin and phenobarbital.

(2) Classification by chemical carcinogens and human tumors

According to the relationship between chemical carcinogens and human tumors, they can be divided into positive carcinogens, suspected carcinogens and potential carcinogens. Affirmative carcinogens are chemical carcinogens that are determined by epidemiological investigations and recognized by clinicians and scientists as having a carcinogenic effect on humans and animals, and which have a dose-response relationship with their carcinogenic effects;

suspected carcinogens have in vitro ability to transform, and the contact time is related to the rate of cancer, and the animal carcinogenic test is positive, but the result is not constant; In addition, such carcinogens lack epidemiological evidence; potential carcinogens generally have some positive results in animal experiments, but there is no data in the population to prove whether they are carcinogenic.

(3) Classified by chemical nature

Chemical carcinogens can be classified into two types: organic chemical carcinogens and inorganic chemical carcinogens. The former is a wide variety, such as most of the compounds in the table. The latter mainly includes carcinogenic metals and metalloids, as well as crystalline silicon and asbestos. Therefore, both exogenous or endogenous chemical carcinogens are dominated by organic chemical carcinogens.

(4). Organic carcinogens

Organic carcinogens can be divided into seven categories:

Polycyclic aromatic hydrocarbons, heterocyclic amines, N-nitroso compounds, dioxins and their analogues, pesticides, azo dyes, bioalkylating agents, triazene compounds, and the like.

(1) Polycyclic aromatic hydrocarbons

Polycyclic aromatic hydrocarbons (PAHs) are a series of polycyclic aromatic hydrocarbon compounds produced by the pyrolysis or incomplete combustion of coal, petroleum, coal tar, tobacco and some organic compounds, many of which are carcinogenic. It is the most widely distributed environmental carcinogen. A large number of investigations and studies in recent years have shown that air, soil, water and plants are contaminated with polycyclic aromatic hydrocarbons. Moreover, modern vehicles, such as automobiles and airplanes, also contain a considerable amount of polycyclic aromatic hydrocarbons in the exhaust gas. Therefore, in the streets with frequent traffic, the pollution of polycyclic aromatic hydrocarbons is also quite serious. **With the development of industry, the problem of carcinogenic polycyclic aromatic hydrocarbons has become a growing concern. It is also the closest environmental carcinogen to humans.**

Certain activities and certain hobbies in human daily life are often closely related to the production of polycyclic aromatic hydrocarbons.

For example, smoking is an important way to produce polycyclic aromatic hydrocarbons, which has been proven to be an important factor in inducing human lung cancer in recent years; another example is the production of carcinogenic polycyclic aromatic hydrocarbons in the cooking, roasting, and smoking of oily foods, and is considered to be one of the main reasons for the increase in gastric cancer rate in some areas. Therefore, polycyclic aromatic hydrocarbons (PAHs) are carcinogens that are the most widely distributed, closely related to humans, and pose a great threat to human health. We must pay sufficient attention to them. In 1973, the International Cancer Research Center (IARC) expert group evaluated that some polycyclic aromatic hydrocarbons are harmful to humans.

(5). Sources of environmental pollution

Natural polycyclic aromatic hydrocarbons are mainly found in coal, petroleum, shale oil, tar, and asphalt. Polycyclic aromatic hydrocarbons can also be produced in the combustion of hydrocarbon-containing materials.

Among the polycyclic aromatic hydrocarbon compounds, the study of benzo[a]pyrene is the most detailed and in-depth, and a relatively accurate measurement method has been established, and it is a substance having a strong carcinogenic effect in polycyclic aromatic hydrocarbons. Therefore, the following mainly uses benzoquinone [a] oxime as an example to illustrate the environmental pollution of this type of chemical substances.

1). Pollution to the atmosphere

The outdoor atmosphere can be contaminated by fixed sources of pollution (such as thermal power stations, industries, enterprises) and mobile sources of pollution (such as aircraft, automobiles, etc.). Especially for cars and trains, the level of pollutants discharged is very low, very close to the breathing zone of people, and often close to residential areas, so sometimes it causes serious pollution. Most of the polycyclic aromatic hydrocarbons adhere to the dust in a crystalline state, and a large amount of air is taken up during the measurement, and a certain amount of dust is filtered and then measured. According to historical data, the highest concentration of benzoquinone [a] in the atmosphere is London, England. <u>The exhaust gas from automobile internal combustion engines must contain polycyclic aromatic hydrocarbon carcinogens.</u>

2). Pollution of the soil

There are many types of polycyclic aromatic hydrocarbons in the soil. For example, rural soils in the eastern United States contain benzo[a]pyrene, phenanthrene, anthracene, anthracene, and valence.

Different chemical companies have different pollutions to the surrounding soil. Some soils containing 200 mg of polycyclic aromatic hydrocarbons per kilogram of soil have been measured in the soil adjacent to the oil plant. It is up to 650 mg per kilogram in the vicinity of the coal tar plant. It has been reported in France that benzo[a]pyrene carcinogens have been isolated from limestone 50 meters below the deep formation.

3). Pollution of water

The water environment includes surface water (rivers, rivers, lakes, reservoirs and oceans) and groundwater, including the most noticeable surface water in residential areas. Dozens of polycyclic aromatic hydrocarbons have been detected from surface water, of which seven or eight are carcinogenic, such as benzopyrene, benzopyrene, dibenzopyrene, quinone, anthracene, benzo[a]pyrene.

4). Pollution of food

Foods also contain a variety of polycyclic aromatic hydrocarbons, such as hydrazine, benzopyrene, dibenzopyrene, benzo[a]pyrene and the like. **Since benzo[a]pyrene is an important component in tobacco, a certain amount of benzo[a]pyrene can often be detected in smoked foods.**

The main sources of benzo[a]pyrene in food are:

a. Bio-synthesis or In vivo synthesis

Benzo[a]pyrene was detected in both unpolluted marine aquatic plants in the Greenland Gulf and in terrestrial plants in mountainous areas far from contaminated areas. Moreover, the content is sometimes similar to the contaminated area, indicating the possibility of synthesizing polycyclic aromatic hydrocarbons in the living body.

b. Absorption and enrichment from contaminated soil and waters

For example, in the contaminated soil, the potatoes and wheat containing benzo[a]pyrene are higher. The content of benzo[a]pyrene in aquatic plants and small plankton is directly related to the content of river water. The benzo[a]pyrene content of plankton in downstream polluted river water is several times higher than that in the upstream clean area. Marine organisms have the ability to enrich polycyclic aromatic hydrocarbons, and marine fish contain benzo[a]pyrene up to 2 to 65 micrograms per kilogram.

Plant foliage is contaminated by atmospheric deposition.

Animal foods also contain polycyclic aromatic hydrocarbons.

c. Pollution during food processing and storage

For food additives and packaging, the bio-vegetable oil is not mechanically pressed, but an organic solvent such as ethane is added to extract the oil. At this time, the organic solvent added may be brought into the vegetable oil if it contains polycyclic aromatic hydrocarbons.

Further, as the paraffin wax applied on the wrapping paper, the polycyclic aromatic hydrocarbon contained therein may contaminate the packaged food.

Processes such as smoking, grilling, and baking, or directly smoking polycyclic aromatic hydrocarbon-containing smoke onto foods, or converting carbohydrates or fats in foods into polycyclic aromatic hydrocarbons due to high temperatures can cause to produce it,.

What is the amount of polycyclic aromatic hydrocarbons that a person consumes from food every day?

It has been estimated that Germans ingest 0.3 micrograms of carcinogenic polycyclic aromatic hydrocarbons per day from value oil, and ingest 10 micrograms from grains, potatoes, vegetables and fruits, of which benzo[a]pyrene accounts for about 3% to 50%.

Therefore, the possible sources of exposure (non-occupational exposure) of PAHs in the general population are as follows:

a. *Contaminated atmosphere (mainly released from wood, coal, mineral oil for automobiles, factories and residents);*

b. *Contaminated indoor air (the main source of release is open furnace and cigarette smoke);*

c. *Smoking;*

d. *Use products containing polycyclic aromatic hydrocarbons;*

e. *Dust inside the house;*

f. *Absorbed from contaminated soil and water through the skin;*

g. *Contaminated food and drinking water.*

5). Carcinogenic mechanism of polycyclic aromatic hydrocarbons

As early as the 1940s, Schmide noticed the relationship between the carcinogenic activity of polycyclic aromatic hydrocarbons and electrical properties. *Later, many people proposed different models to explain the structure and activity of polycyclic aromatic hydrocarbons, which are briefly described below. The carcinogenic mechanism of carcinogens in the body is still poorly understood.*

6. N-nitroso compounds

N-nitroso compounds (NOC) are widely found in nature, and humans are mainly absorbed into the body through diet, drinking water and the like. N-nitroso compounds are a class of organic compounds with similar structures. The gastric cancer caused by it has been widely verified in animal experiments. Therefore, whether human gastric cancer is related to this has become an issue of epidemiological concern. By 1983, more than 300 nitroso compounds had been studied, 90% of which were carcinogenic.

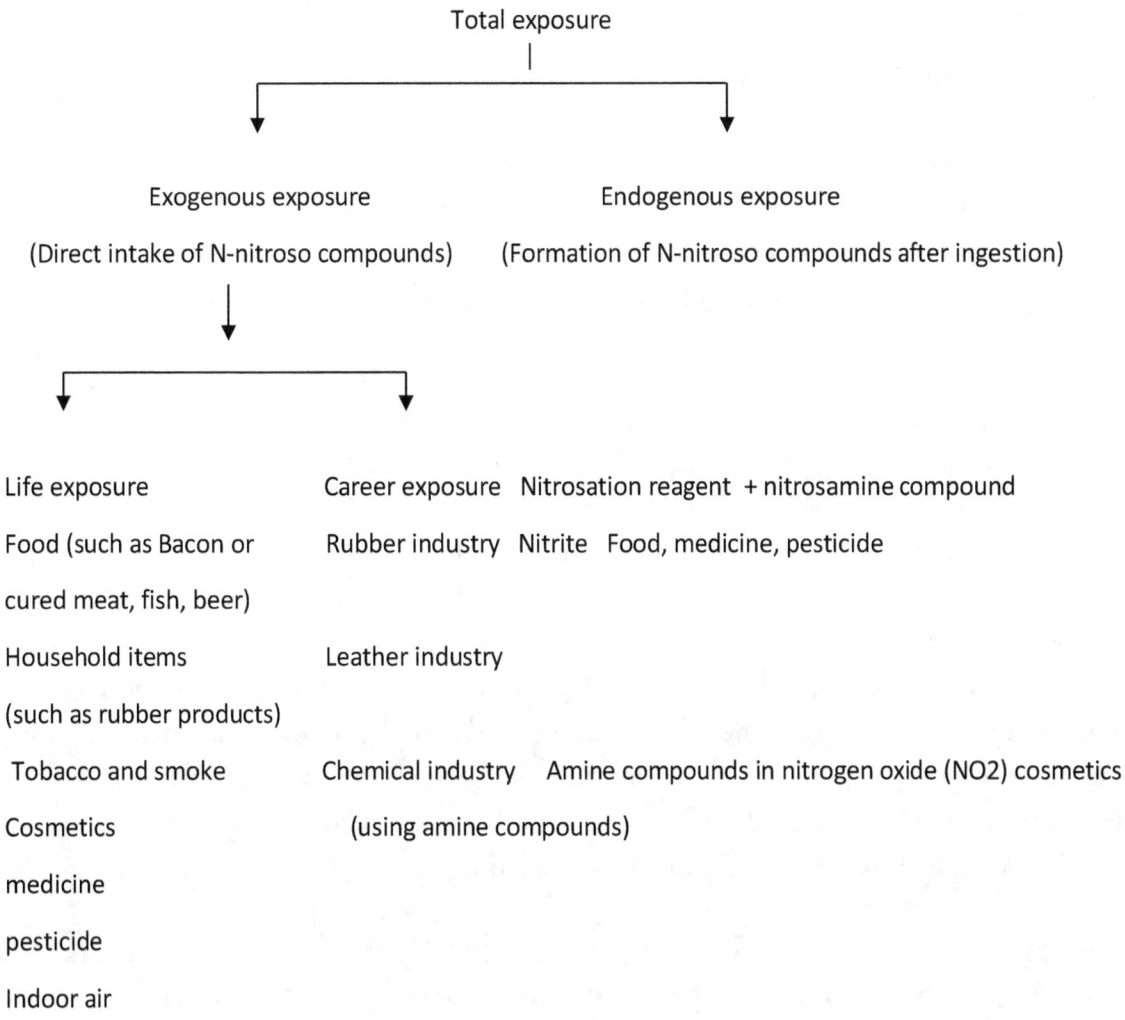

Figure Human contact with N-nitroso compounds

(1) Sources of N-nitroso compounds in the environment

Human contact with N-nitroso compounds in the environment, and Wang Liansheng et al. made a detailed summary. There are two types: external exposure and endogenous exposure. Exogenous exposure refers to the direct intake of N-nitroso compounds from the environment, and can be divided into two categories: life exposure and occupational exposure; Endogenous exposure refers to the reaction of nitrosamine compounds present in foods, medicines, and cosmetics with nitrosating agents to form N-nitroso compounds.

(2) N-nitrosamines in foods

A. Marinated smoked meat:

Wang Liansheng and others have systematically analyzed N nitrosamines in 395 commercial meat and meat products in Germany. The results show that only nitrosamine contamination occurs in samples treated with nitrite or nitrate. Among them, salted pork and ham are most polluted by nitrosamines.

Bacon, ham, beef sausage, salami, and meat bread usually do not change their original N-nitrosodimethylamine concentration after frying, but the concentration of N-nitrosopyrrolidine increases.

The main source of N-nitrosopyrrolidine ingested by the British is fried bacon. The situation is similar in the United States and Canada. The content of volatile nitrosamines in raw bacon is very small. The amount of nitrosamines produced during frying is affected by the cooking method, temperature and cooking time. For example, the pyrrolidine nitrosamine produced by frying bacon in a pan is much more than that produced in a microwave oven. The bacon sample did not form pyrrolidine nitrosamine at 99 ° C for 105 minutes. However, pyrrolidine nitrosamine can be produced by frying at 204 ° C for 4 minutes.

<u>Janzowshi et al. studied 33 samples of fried bacon, ham, red sausage and sausage, and found that 9 of them contained non-volatile carcinogen N-nitroso-3-hydroxypyrrolidine. Lee et al. also detected the carcinogen in fried bacon.</u>

B. Fish

Trace amounts of volatile nitrosamines have been found in fish and fish products, and Kawabate et al. conducted a detailed study of an important Japanese food, dried fish, which was cooked in a gasifier. The amount of N-nitrosodimethylamine increased and no N-nitrosopyrrolidine was detected. After the squid is cooked in a gasifier, the amount of N-nitrosodimethylamine increases more, and the cooked whale also contains N-nitrosopyrrolidine. N-nitrosodimethylamine was detected in all fish samples tested.

a. Chinese fish

After marinating with nitrate-containing sodium chloride, N-nitrosodimethylamine can be detected. The content of volatile nitrosamines N-nitrosodimethylamine, N-nitrosodiethylamine and N-nitrosomorpholine in salted Guangzhou fish is very low, an the content will increase after cooking. N-nitroso-N-propylamine and N-nitrosobis-N-butylamine were not detected in the raw fish samples, but were detected in the fish after cooking or cooked.

b. Fish in Western countries contain only a small amount of nitroso carcinogens, and mainly N-nitrosodimethylamine. In the UK, 80% of the 94 samples tested contained nitroso carcinogens. However, most of the content is very low. Similar results have been reported in the United States, Canada, Sweden, and Germany.

C. *Dairy products:*

In some dairy products, such as dry cheese, milk powder, milk wine, etc., trace amounts of volatile nitrosamines are present.

D. *Vegetable and fruit:*

Some vegetables and melons contain amines, nitrates and nitrites. Therefore, when processing vegetables, or it has the long-term storage, amines and nitrites in vegetables and fruits react to form trace amounts of sub- Nitramine.

The incidence of esophageal cancer is high in some areas of China.

A characteristic N-nitroso compound, N-nitroso-N-(3-methylbutyl)-N-methylacetonyl nitrosamine, was found in corn bun in the region.

E. *Beer and other beverages:*

The most surprising finding in Wang Liansheng's research on nitrosamine contamination in food is that beer often contains N-nitrosodimethylamine.

Some European beer is also contaminated. Studies have found that beer is the only source of N-nitrosodimethylamine by ripening. Draft beer will only have a small amount of negligible N-itrosodimethylamine.

Nitrification reagent In the ripening process or curing process (1500~1800 °C), it exists in the form of nitrogen oxides. Improving ripening conditions can significantly reduce the concentration of nitramine in malt beer.

Other alcoholic beverages such as wine, cider, rice wine and spirits are usually free of volatile nitrosamines. Six of the seven tested Scotch whiskies contain N-nitrosodimethylamine; Waller et al. studied 145 French apple brandies and found that 50% of them contained N-nitrosodimethylamine.

(3) Tobacco and smoke

Hoffmann, Brunemann, Hecht and colleagues first studied nitroso compounds in tobacco and smoke. The freshly harvested tobacco does not contain nitrosamines. However, nitrosamines are formed during the drying, aging, and fermentation processes. Nitrosamines can form in smoking, and their formation is related to the amount of nitrate in tobacco.

Tobacco-specific nitrosamines are the only known type of nasal cancer carcinogens. Nitrosamines in snuff can be extracted from tobacco blocks and can also be detected in the saliva of snuff and chew tobacco.

(4) Pesticides

Since Roos et al. have confirmed for the first time that pesticides have been contaminated with nitrosamines, extensive research has been carried out. In the United States, more than 300 compounds were studied. Pesticides containing the following genes have been identified as potential mesogenic carriers:

Dinitroaniline derivatives (especially 2,6-dinitroaniline), dimethylamine salts with phenoxy chain, diethanolamine salts and triethanolamine salts (such as maleic acid hydrazide), quaternary amine compounds in acidic pesticides And morpholine derivatives.

Nitrosamines in pesticides can exist as impurities and can also exist as contaminants. There are several ways to form them:

a. Side reactions during the production process;

b. Contaminated chemicals are used in the synthesis;

c. Use of preservatives (especially nitrites);

d. Nitrosation reagents in the environment;

e. Intermolecular rearrangement.

In addition, many chlorine-containing pesticides can be nitrosated under experimental conditions to form amine precursors of N-nitroso compounds.

The US Environmental Protection Agency has made a decision to reduce human exposure to pesticides that can be derived from nitroso compounds.

As a result, many pesticide manufacturers have reduced or even eliminated nitrosamine contamination in pesticides by preventing nitrosation and direct chemical damage.

(5) Cosmetics

Diethanolamine, triethanolamine and some salts thereof (e.g., lauryl sulfate) are widely used as emulsifiers in the manufacture of many cosmetics (such as ointments, creams, shampoos, lipsticks). Contamination of nitrosamines in cosmetics may be the result of the use of contaminated paints or contact with nitrosating agents such as NO_2 during the manufacturing process. Cosmetics widely used in the United States were analyzed, and N-nitrosodiethanolamine was detected in 27 of 29 samples. Skin contact with N-nitrosodiethanolamine-contaminated cosmetics, N-nitrosodiethanolamine can be detected in the urine, indicating that the complex is easily absorbed through the skin.

(6) Carcinogenic mechanism

The carcinogenic effects of nitrosamines are related to their chemical structure, route of administration, drug dosage and animal species.

Regarding the carcinogenic mechanism of nitrosamines, it is generally believed that nitrosamine compounds can form diazane under the action of mixed functional oxidase and then dealkylate to form a free methyl group. The latter catalyzes the nucleic acid and proteination of cells, especially the guanine of RNA and DNA. **The alkylation of the nucleic acid changes the genetic characteristics of the cell, and the tumor occurs by somatic mutation or abnormal cell differentiation.**

For nitrosamides, it is generally considered that it can cause cancer directly.

The incidence of esophageal cancer is quite high in parts of China, South Africa and Iran. Chinese scientists have revealed **the relationship between the incidence of esophageal cancer and nitroso amino acids in the urine, including nitroso-sarcosine. And Nitrosylsarcosine is a carcinogen for esophageal cancer.** In high-risk areas of esophageal cancer in China, the potential danger of endogenous nitrosylation is also high. In China and South Africa, **nitrosamine contamination in moldy foods has been considered a cause** or an **incentive of esophageal cancer.** In the south of China, nasopharyngeal carcinoma is more common. The studies have shown that its incidence is related to nitrosoproline, and salted fish with more intake is an important pathogenic factor or ingestion of more salted fish is an important cause of disease. Nitrosamines such as N-nitrosodimethylamine can be detected in steamed salted fish. Feeding rats with Guangdong salted fish can induce nasal cancer. These tests prove that nitrosamine is the causative agent of nasopharyngeal carcinoma.

Nitrate and nitrite in foods such as fish and meat:

Salting fish and meat is an ancient method. Its efficacy is the reduction of nitrate to nitrite by bacteria. Nitrite can inhibit the growth of some spoilage bacteria, thus achieving the purpose of preservation. About 50 years ago, it was found that only a small amount of nitrite was used to treat food, and a large amount of nitrate was achieved. The nitrite gradually replaces the nitrate as a preservative and colorant. The amount of residues in the provisional meat products in China shall not exceed 30 g/kg for sodium nitrite, and the canned meat shall not exceed 50 g/kg.

Amines in the environment

Nitrite and nitrate are abundantly present in nature, and secondary amines (secondary amines) may also be present. Nitrite and secondary amines are not carcinogenic, but nitrosamines can be biosynthesized under acidic conditions.

Gastric cancer is one of the common multiple malignancies. The cause of gastric cancer may be related to the level of nitrate and nitrite in the environment, especially the amount of nitrate in drinking water.

According to the etiology of esophageal cancer, the incidence of esophageal cancer is related to environmental factors.

In environmental factors that cause liver cancer, in addition to aflatoxin, soil nitrogen and nitrosamines may be important environmental factors. Non-staple foods in high-incidence areas of *liver cancer*, especially pickles contain nitrosamines. The determination of nitrosamines in pickles in high-incidence areas of liver cancer shows that the detection rate of nitrosamines is as high as 60%. From the results of epidemiological investigations at home and abroad, certain cancers in humans may be associated with N-nitroso compounds.

Chile's saltpeter production ranks first in the world. The use of nitrate fertilizers in agriculture makes the nitrite content in foods high and the chance of synthesizing nitramine in the body increases. Therefore, it is believed that Chilean gastric cancer mortality ranks first in the world. Linzhou City in Henan Province in China is also one of the world's high incidence areas of esophageal cancer. It has successfully induced esophageal cancer in rats with high-yield sauerkraut soup concentrate or sauerkraut extract.

A large amount of evidence indicates that N-nitroso compounds are carcinogenic causes of various cancers in the human body, including oral cancer, lung cancer, esophageal cancer, pancreatic cancer, liver cancer, nasopharyngeal cancer and bladder cancer.

7. Measures to prevent the harm of nitroso compounds

The nitrosylation process of nitroso compounds can be affected by a variety of compounds and environmental conditions such as vitamin C, vitamin E, citric acid and phenolic compounds can inhibit the synthesis.

Sucrose blocks the synthesis of nitroso compounds at a pH of 3, and its blocking effect is good when its molecular concentration is twice that of nitrite. In the preparation of sausages, the addition of vitamin C at the same time as the addition of nitrite prevents the formation of dimethyl nitrosamines. However, vitamin C has no effect on the formed nitrosamines. Chen Bingqing et al. summarized the following measures to prevent the harm of nitroso compounds:

<u>**(1) to ensure that food is fresh, which is important to reduce the content of nitroso compounds in food**</u>. Preventing food poisoning can prevent the contamination of other microorganisms, because some bacteria can reduce nitrate to nitrite and decompose proteins.

The default is an amine compound, and there is also enzymatic nitrosylation. Therefore, food should be kept fresh during food processing; prevent microbial contamination.

(2) Prevent and mitigate the harm of nitroso compounds through diet, vitamin C can block the process of nitrosation in the stomach

a. Vitamin C is effective both in vivo and in vitro in inhibiting the formation of nitrosamines by precursors. Vitamin C can block the synthesis of nitrosamines in the stomach and reduce the exposure level of nitrosamines in the stomach, which is manifested by a decrease in the content of nitrosamines in the gastric juice.

b. Some natural juices also contain unknown ingredients other than ascorbic acid that inhibit nitrosylation.

c. Soy products can also effectively inhibit the synthesis of N-nitrous oxide. The order of inhibition is soybean milk powder > bean paste > tofu, soy products can reduce the nitrite content and induce liver cancer with obvious preventive effect.

d. The antioxidant effect of tea in the body is not single. It is not only can the self-suppressing base be directly eliminated, but also the prevalence of free radical scavenging can be eliminated and it is inhibiting the comprehensive process of carcinogen activation and promotion of carcinogen degradation and sewage in activated state and blocking lipid peroxidation and It inhibits peroxidative damage and thus plays a role in preventing cancer.

e. Chinese scholars have found that garlic and allicin can inhibit nitrate-reducing bacteria in the stomach, and the amount of nitrite in the stomach is significantly reduced.

f. In addition, kiwifruit and seabuckthorn juice also have a blocking effect, and the former also inhibits the mutagenic effect of N-nitrosodimethylamine.

3) Strictly control the food processing process

It is to minimize the use of nitrates and nitrites so as to reduce the amount of nitrosated precursor. When the processing technology is feasible, try to use nitrite and nitrate substitutes.

Dioxins and their analogues

Since January 1999, **countries such as Belgium, the Netherlands, and France have been contaminated with dioxin, which has led to high levels of carcinogens, dioxin, in poultry, livestock and dairy products. After the incident, it has aroused widespread concern in all countries of the world.**

The fly ash produced by urban fixed waste incineration contains dioxin. Incineration of waste containing polyvinyl chloride may be higher.

Automobile exhaust

Due to the incomplete combustion of gasoline, car exhaust can release dioxins.

In industrialized countries, dioxins are mainly from municipal solid waste incineration, impurities in chlorine-containing chemicals, pulp bleaching and vehicle exhaust emissions. China has a different source of pollution than industrialized countries. Due to the need for schistosomiasis prevention, a large amount of PCP-Na is used to eliminate snails, which causes serious pollution of rivers and lakes in the Yangtze River basin in China. In addition, small paper mills are scattered throughout China, and the discharged wastewater and waste slag cause serious pollution of major rivers and lakes. Therefore, the pollution of dioxin industry in China must not be ignored.

(1) The way of dioxin enters the human body

The human body can be exposed to dioxins in different ways, including food, air, and drinking water. Of these, 90% comes from diet, and animal food is its main source. In theory, the removal of fat from meat, the use of low-fat milk powder, and the intake of vegetables, fruits, and grains can effectively prevent the harm of dioxins to humans.

(2) Food contamination pathways

Due to the fat solubility of dioxins and their stability in the environment, and environmental pollution caused by the production and use of chlorine-containing chemicals, the incineration of fixed waste, and the bleaching process during papermaking, most of them are in water body and through the food chain process of aquatic plants, zooplankton---- herbivores fish---Fish-eating fish and Goose and duck, and other poultry, and enriched in fish and poultry and their proteins. Simultaneously, **due to the flow of the ambient atmosphere, the dioxin in the**

fly ash settles on the ground plants, polluts vegetables, food and feed. Animals contaminated feed also cause accumulation of dioxins. Therefore, fish, poultry, their eggs, and meat have become the main contaminated foods.

(3) Carcinogenicity

2,3,7,8-tetrachlorodibenzo-p-dioxin is highly carcinogenic to animals.

Nineteen studies in four animal species (rats, mice, hamsters, and fish) all showed positive results. Continuously 2,3,7,8-tetrachlorodibenzo-pair Dioxin Pollution or contamination on Rodent can induce multiple sites of tumor on both sexes. The low dose of causing liver cancer in mice is as low as 10 pg/g (body weight). Epidemiological studies suggest that population exposure to 2,3,7,8-tetrachlorodibenzo-p-dioxin and its homologues is associated with an overall increased risk of all cancers in the population. **According to this, the International Center for Cancer Research identified it as a Class I carcinogen that is carcinogenic to humans in 1997.**

Dioxin is a whole or entire carcinogen and can cause cancer by itself. Dioxins can be considered human carcinogens based on animal experiments and epidemiological studies.

The International Agency for Research on Cancer has classified it as a recognized human carcinogen (Class I).

(4) Control measures for dioxins

In the face of the harm caused by dioxin pollution, based on the investigation and research of the major industrialized countries in the world, it has developed measures to prevent dioxin pollution, in combination with China's special national conditions, the following recommendations are proposed for China's dioxin control:

1). Strengthen the treatment of waste incineration and control emissions

Control measures are set by the National Environmental Protection Agency to reduce emissions of dioxins in large incineration plants.

2). Improve the production process and reduce the production of dioxin

Control dioxin produces during the production of chemical products to prevent environmental pollution.

3). Expand the promotion or propaganda of environmental protection and food hygiene

Most of the dioxin that comes into contact with humans comes from meals. Therefore, the safety of the food supply system is crucial. In theory, paying attention to the dietary structure and reducing the intake of animal fat can reduce the intake of dioxins. Fibrous foods and chlorophyll help eliminate long-term accumulation of dioxins in the body.

However, in order to solve the problem completely, It is necessary to raise the overall level of human understanding and production capacity, focus on ecological construction, reduce environmental pollution and achieve the goal of modernization, in order to ensure the sustainable, stable and healthy development of human society.

Gathering wisdom, conquering cancer

- for the benefit of mankind

Second

How to prevent cancer? I see two

(1) Finding problems and asking questions from follow-up results

(One)

Finding problems and asking questions from follow-up results (Hint: Studying postoperative recurrence and prevention of metastasis is the key to improving long-term outcomes after surgery)

Navigate

(To overcome cancer, where is the road? How can the road be found?)

↓

Pathfinding and footprinting

(the research and scientific research results and the scientific and technological innovation series of anti-cancer, anti-cancer metastasis)

Create the research institute of the environmental protection and cancer prevention and carry out cancer prevention system engineering

↓

Published cancer monographs

(3 Chinese editions are published nationwide, 4 full English editions are published worldwide)

↓

Participate in the International Oncology Conference
(Participate in the AACR Academic Conference, Washington)

↓

Visiting the Stirling Cancer Institute in Houston, USA (2009)

↓

Walking out of the new level of immune regulation molecule level

---------*it has gone out of a new road to overcome cancer*

---------*it is Published the English monograph "The Road to Overcome Cancer" in December 6, 2016, published in Washington, DC, worldwide.*

(2) XZ-C proposes to conquer cancer and launch a general attack

(Two)

XZ-C proposes to conquer cancer and launch a general attack

Xu Ze proposes to "to conquer cancer and launch the general attack of cancer" in Chapter 38 of "New Concepts and New Methods for Cancer Treatment" (Beijing Publishing, 2011), which is the first time in the world.

1. What is the total attack on cancer?

The general attack is to carry out the three-stage work of cancer prevention, cancer control and cancer treatment in the whole process of cancer occurrence and development, and carry out the simultaneous and simultaneous prevention and treatment.

What is cancer prevention, cancer control, and cancer treatment?

Namely:

cancer prevention - before cancer formation

cancer control - precancerous lesions with malignant tendencies

treating cancer - has formed a cancerous foci or metastasis

Change the current hospital mode

Change current treatment mode

Namely:

change the current hospital-oriented mode

change the current treatment mode focusing on the middle and late stages of treatment

change only the treatment without defense, change into the defense, control, and treatment at the same time

How to implement this new mode of running a hospital?

It is necessary to establish a hospital for prevention, control and treatment according to the whole process of cancer occurrence and development.

2, the way out of cancer treatment in the "three early" (early detection, early diagnosis, early treatment)

Early cancer treatment is good, can heal, especially precancerous lesions, well treated, can be cured.

Create the research institute of the environmental protection and cancer prevention and carry out cancer prevention system engineering

(3) XZ-C proposes to create the science city as the research bases of conquering cancer research bases

(three)

XZ-C proposes to overcome the general attack of cancer and create a cancer science city, which is the first time in the world.

In order to overcome cancer, it is necessary to create a science city that overcomes the general attack of cancer.

How to overcome cancer, I see it 1 - 5

1. How to overcome cancer? To overcome cancer, we must create the Innovative Molecular Oncology School.

(1) Why does it need to build the "Innovative Molecular Oncology Medical School"?

(2) How to establish the "Innovative Molecular Oncology Medical School"?

2. How to overcome cancer? In order to overcome cancer, it must create "innovative molecular tumor occurrence, development, prevention and treatment of hospitals"(Global demonstration of occurrence, development, full-scale prevention and treatment of hospitals)

(1) Why does it need to build? (2) How to create?

3. How to overcome cancer? In order to overcome cancer, we must create the Innovative Molecular Oncology Institute.

(1) Why does it need to start to build? (2) How to create?

4. How to overcome cancer? In order to overcome cancer, the Experimental Medicine Cancer Animal Experimental Center must be created.

(1) Why does it need to build ? (2) How to create?

5. How to overcome cancer?

In order to overcome cancer, we must create "Innovative Molecular Tumor Pharmaceuticals" and "Create Research Group and Laboratory for the Analysis of Active Components, Molecular Weight, Structural Formula, Immunopharmacology at the Molecular Level of anti-cancer and anti-cancer metastasis Chinese medications"

(1) Why does it need to start to build up?

Because conquering cancer requires research and development of effective drugs for anti-cancer and anti-cancer metastasis, XZ-C believes that two wheels must be used to overcome cancer:

One is the life science, biomedical (modern medicine) A wheel.

One is the clinical basis, immune regulation, anti-cancer (Chinese herbal medicine) B wheel.

Its purpose is:

It is in-depth development of effective Chinese herbal medicine with anti-cancer, anti-metastatic from Chinese medications, and it to remove the crude and keep the marrow as storage, and it is to be natural medicine and Chinese herbal medicine as a resource for modern research, making precision medicine.

It is to further experimental study on the molecular level of immunomodulatory anti-cancer Chinese medicine.

It is to further explore the cancer prevention and anti-cancer Chinese herbal medicines for the prevention and treatment of early carcinoma in situ and precancerous lesions.

(4) XZ-C proposes to create the research institute of cancer prevention and the cancer prevention system engineering

XZ-C proposes that to overcome cancer and to launch the general attack on cancer must establish the Cancer Prevention Research Institute and the cancer prevention system project. This is the first time to be proposed in the world.

To conduct anti-cancer research, find cancer-causing factors, detect the source of carcinogens or carcinogenic factors, and try to prevent the damage of these carcinogenic factors to the human body; the Cancer Research Institute should conduct anti-cancer research, and there is many and wide things or contents which are needed for research.

To track the source of carcinogens or carcinogenic factors.

In the search for the cause and condition of cancer, the most prominent thing is that more than 90% of cancers are caused by environmental factors.

1. Relationship between air pollution and cancer

Humans have developed tens of millions of tons of coal, oil and natural gas as fuel and energy. In the production and life processes such as thermal power generation, smelting steel, automobiles, airplanes, and household fuels, **a large amount of tar, bituminous coal, dust and other harmful substances are discharged into the atmosphere around the clock, causing air pollution.**

Air pollution can cause many diseases, especially respiratory diseases, the most serious is lung cancer.

2, water pollution and cancer

The pollution of water quality is mainly caused by industrial and agricultural production and urban sewage. There are many types of pollutants in water. Pesticides and Insecticides are one of the important pollutants in water bodies. Surfactants in neutral detergents also have a cancer-promoting effect.

3. Soil pollution and cancer

A large amount of industrial waste water residue and pesticides and fertilizers are injected into the soil, **which deteriorates soil quality and accumulates poisons, posing a threat to human health and are a carcinogenic factor.**

4. Chemistry and cancer

5. Physical factors and cancer

6. Biological factors and cancer

7. Diet and cancer

8. Lifestyle and cancer

9. Clothing, food, housing, travel, house decoration, etc. and cancer

The way in which so many carcinogens or carcinogenic factors should be studied.

It is to study these sources of pollution and try to stop at the source.

It is to study these carcinogenic mechanisms and their carcinogenic effects.

It is to study how to reduce or prevent these carcinogens.

Because cancer patients cover the whole world, the pollution of industrial and agricultural wastewater, waste residue and waste gas also covers the whole world. Therefore, it is necessary to globally attack the cancer attack. Therefore, it must work together globally to conquer the cancer and to launch the general attack.

Professor Xu Ze suggested:

1). All countries, provinces and states should establish cancer prevention research institutes (or institutions), carry out cancer prevention system projects, and carry out cancer prevention work for their own country, province and city.

2). Countries establish cancer prevention regulations and carry out comprehensively (some should be legislated)

3). I will use this project to recommend the World Health Organization to hold an cancer prevention campaign, with the goal of reducing the incidence of cancer.

Conquering cancer is a frontier of science and a worldwide problem. Cancer is a human disaster, covering the whole world. People all over the world are eager to hope that one day they can overcome cancer and benefit mankind.

Cancer is a disaster for all mankind, and it must fight globally.

The global people struggle together

Conquering cancer and launching a general attack, this is an unprecedented event for the benefit of mankind.

(5) Cancer prevention research work cannot walk slowly and it should run forward and save the wounded

(Fives)

The research work of prevention of cancer cannot walk slowly and should run ahead and save the wounded

Why did I propose to overcome cancer and launch a general attack?

It is because I have been working on the research and design of cancer series for 5-6 years and we have made a complete set of basic ideas and designs, plans and blueprints to overcome cancer.

And in the entire chapter 38 in "New Concepts and New Methods for Cancer Treatment" published in 2011 it was to put forward the "strategic ideas and recommendations for conquering cancer" and it was proposed "to overcome conquer and launch the general attack of cancer."

Later, in 2013, it was proposed "To build a comprehensive design for the Cancer Science City". In August 2013, it was first proposed internationally: "XZ-C Scientific Research Plan for Overcoming cancer and launching the General Attack of Cancer". It was proposed in July 2015 and named "Dawning C-type plan". It was put forward "to overcome cancer and to launch the general attack of cancer" and "to build a science city to overcome cancer", this work is being reported and pleasing to implement.

Conquering cancer and launching the general attack of cancer is an unprecedented work of humanity. It is necessary to personally create experience and practice it personally.

About 8,550 people in China are diagnosed with cancer every day, and 6 people are diagnosed with cancer every minute.

Therefore, scientific research work that do research to overcome cancer and to launch the general attack of cancer cannot walk slowly and should run forward to save the wounded.

2017.2.5 Reference message

[Effie, Geneva, February 3rd]

The World Health Organization released data on the occasion of the "World Cancer Day" on February 4th. At present, 8.8 million people die of cancer every year in the world, and among them the number of deaths from respiratory cancer is the highest, reaching 1.695 million per year.

The latest data is based on 2015 statistics, increasing the number of people dying from cancer each year from an estimated 8.1 million in 2010 to 8.8 million.

The most deadly cancers that are second only to respiratory cancer are liver cancer (788,000 deaths per year), colorectal cancer (774,000), stomach cancer (753,300) and breast cancer (571,000).

Cancers such as esophageal cancer (415,000), pancreatic cancer (358,000), prostate cancer (334,800), and lymphoma (334,300) also have high mortality rates worldwide.

In terms of gender, there are nearly 5 million male deaths among 8.8 million cancer deaths.

For men, the most common types of cancers are respiratory cancer and liver cancer.

For women, the cancer with the highest mortality rate is breast cancer and respiratory cancer.

In terms of regional distribution, the most common cancer cases are in the western Pacific, with respiratory cancer and liver cancer accounting for the highest proportion.

Second only to the Western Pacific is Southeast Asia, where respiratory cancer, oral cancer and throat cancer account for the highest proportion.

In Europe, the most common cancer is respiratory cancer, followed by colorectal cancer.

The disaster of cancer covers the whole world. People all over the world are eager to hope to overcome cancer one day. It is hoped that the state, government, experts, scholars and scientists can find out cancer prevention measures so that people can stay away from cancer.

Create the research institute of the environmental protection and cancer prevention and carry out cancer prevention system engineering

Professor Xu Ze has been engaged in clinical surgery for 60 years.

It has been 30 years since the basic research and clinical validation of animal experiments to overcome cancer. I deeply understand that cancer should not only pay attention to treatment, but also pay attention to prevention, so as to stop cancer at the source. So it is proposed:

It should be launched to conquer cancer and to launch the general attack of cancer, prevention and treatment are equally important.

1. **How to overcome cancer?**

<u>Its purpose should be:</u>

(1)

1), reduce the incidence of cancer

2), improve the cure rate of cancer, prolong the survival of cancer patients and improve the quality of life

(2) reach:

1/3 can prevent

1/3 can be cured

1/3 can prolong life through treatment

2. <u>**How to improve the cure rate?**</u>

How to cure or to treat?

<u>It should go out of a new way to cure cancer:</u>

(1) Conquer cancer and launch a general attack

1). The general attack is to carry out the three-stage work of cancer prevention, cancer control and cancer treatment in the whole process of cancer occurrence and development, and carry out simultaneously three carriages, go hand in hand, and drive together.

2). Change the current mode of running a hospital—that is, change the current mode of running a hospital with a focus on treatment.

Change the current treatment mode - that is, change the current treatment mode focusing on the middle and late stages of treatment, and change the treatment only to prevention, control, and treatment at the same important level.

(2) How to implement this new mode of running a hospital?

It is necessary to establish a hospital for prevention, control and treatment according to the whole process of cancer occurrence and development.

(3) The way out for cancer treatment is "three early" (early detection, early diagnosis, early treatment), early cancer treatment is effective, can be cured, especially cancer lesions, well treated, can be cured.

3. How to reduce the incidence of cancer?

How to prevent?

It should go out of a new way to prevent cancer:

(1) XZ-C thinks:

How to prevent cancer? An anti-cancer research institute should be created and cancer prevention system project should be created. It should study carcinogenic factors and their sources, and study to try to stop or avoid them.

(2) What to prevent?

a. What are the carcinogenic factors?

b. What are the sources of carcinogenic factors?

How to prevent it?

a, how to reduce its source

b, how to stop its source

Cancer prevention work should be blocked at the source and should prevent the source of carcinogenic factors.

Cancer prevention is active, it is attack

Cancer treatment is passive, it is abiding

How to prevent? What to prevent? How to prevent it?

It should be studied in depth, the evaluation goal is: reduce the incidence rate

How to cure? What to cure? How to cure?

It should be studied in depth, the evaluation goal is: improve the cure rate

(6) The research work of how to improve the cure rate of cancer

(Six)

How to improve the cure rate of cancer? How to prolong the survival of cancer patients, improve the quality of life and reduce complications

1. <u>How to cure?</u>

After more than 30 years of experimental and clinical validation studies, we have embarked on the new path to overcome cancer.

(1) Through experimental research and anti-cancer research of Chinese medicine immunopharmacology and the combination of Chinese and Western medicine on the molecular level, <u>we have taken out the new path of a traditional Chinese medicine immune regulation</u>, regulate immune activity, prevent thymus atrophy, promote thymic hyperplasia, protect bone marrow hematopoietic function, and improve immune surveillance at the molecular level of the combination with Western medicine and Chinese medicine to overcome cancer.

We have initially embarked on the road of overcoming cancer with an XZ-C immune regulation, and the molecular level of the combination of Chinese and Western -----the "Chinese-style anti-cancer" new road.

a, I am a clinical surgeon, for chest surgery work and general surgery work, why do I study cancer?

This is due to the results of a petition to a group of cancer patients after surgery:

Since 1985, I have conducted a petition to more than 3,000 patients with postoperative thoracic and abdominal cancer. I found that most patients relapsed or metastasized within 2-3 years after surgery.

From the follow-up results it was found:

Postoperative recurrence and metastasis are the key factors affecting long-term outcomes.

Therefore, it also raised an important question for us:

That is, clinicians must pay attention to and study the prevention and treatment of postoperative recurrence and metastasis to improve the long-term efficacy after surgery.

So we established an experimental surgery laboratory to conduct experimental tumor research:

Cancer cell transplantation was performed, a tumor animal model was established, and a series of experimental tumor studies were carried out.

b. We have conducted a full-scale clinical research work in the laboratory for 4 years, which is a basic clinical study.

From the experimental results, it was found that the host thymus was acutely atrophied after inoculation of cancer cells, cell proliferation was blocked, and the volume was significantly reduced.

From the above experimental studies, it is found that thymus atrophy and low immune function may be one of the causes and pathogenesis of cancer. So the hint:

Its (cancer) treatment principle must be to try to prevent thymus atrophy, promote thymocyte proliferation, and boost immunity.

In order to try to prevent thymus atrophy, promote thymocyte proliferation, and increase immunity, we look for both Chinese medicine and western medicine.

The existing medicines of that western medicine can improve immunity and promote the proliferation of thymus are rare or few or there are few existing western medicine which can improve immunity and promote the proliferation of thymus. So we changed to look for Chinese herbal medicine.

Why was it to have been looking for drugs that promote thymic hyperplasia, prevent thymus atrophy, and boost immunity from traditional Chinese medicine?

It is because within the polysaccharides Chinese medicine and tonic Chinese medicine of Chinese herbal medicine, many of them have the role of regulating immunity.

Research on anti-cancer immunity of Chinese medicine polysaccharides is progressing rapidly. A large number of immunopharmacological studies have been carried out at the molecular level, and polysaccharides can improve the body's immune surveillance system.

In our laboratory a series of experimental studies have been carried out to find new anti-cancer Chinese medicine with anti-cancer, anti-metastasis, stopping Thymus atrophy, and increasing immune-regulation.

c. **A series products of XZ-C immune regulation and control anti-cancer Chinese medicine through the exclusive scientific research and development**

a). Experimental study + clinical application + typical case + case list

b.) Self-developed XZ-C (XU ZE-China) (Xu Ze - China) immune regulation and control anti-cancer series of traditional Chinese medicine preparations

They are developed from experimental research to clinical verification, it has been applied to clinical practice on the basis of the success of animal experiments. After more than 12,000 clinical trials in more than 20 years, the curative effect is remarkable and it is independent innovation.

XZ-C immunomodulation anticancer Chinese medicine is developed from more than 200 traditional Chinese herbal medicines in China, in which 48 kinds of Chinese herbal medicines with good tumor inhibition rate were screened by anti-tumor experiments in cancer-bearing mice.

After compounding the compound, the tumor-inhibiting experiment was carried out in the cancer-bearing mice, and the compound tumor inhibition rate was much higher than that of the single-flavor drug.

Among them, XZ-C1 inhibits cancer cells 100%, does not kill normal cells, and has the effect of strengthening the body and improving the immune function of the human body.

The pharmacodynamic study of XZ-C from our experiments proves that it has a good tumor inhibition rate for Ehrlich ascites carcinoma, S180 and H22 hepatocellular carcinoma.

Acute toxicity test in mice showed no obvious side effects. In the clinical long-term oral administration for several years (2-6-8 years), no obvious side effects were observed.

Middle and advanced cancer patients are mostly weak and weak, fatigue, lack of appetite, after taking XZ-C immune regulation and control anti-cancer Chinese medicine for 4-8-12 weeks, the patients can significantly improve appetite, sleep, relieve pain, and gradually restore physical strength.

Why do I want to propose prevent cancer?

Professor Xu Ze proposed that research on cancer prevention must be emphasized in order to overcome cancer. Because the treatment of the disease first studies the cause and treats the cause, it can be effective. Cancer prevention also first studies the carcinogenic factors and their sources. Aiming at the carcinogenic factors to stop, it can be effective.

It is believed that it is not only relying on the existing cancer prevention popularization knowledge, but also on macro, micro, ultra-micro and high-tech research.

<u>**How to conduct cancer research?**</u>

<u>**Professor Xu Ze proposed:**</u>

<u>**Create a cancer prevention research institute and create a cancer prevention research system project and establish a graduate school.**</u>

Academic committee, expert, scholar of "Science City for Overcoming the General Attack of Cancer" will lead 100 doctoral and postgraduate students to conduct research on cancer prevention and cancer prevention. I will draw up a large number of in-depth research topics, based on known science, to explore future science, and to develop science.

Now is the fourth stage of our research work. After 2011, it is being carried out and proceeded, doing research work, Step by step in-depth and positioning research goals or "targets" to reduce cancer incidence, improving the cure rate and prolonging the survival period.

We have been working on cancer research for 28 years:

The first three stages of experimental research and clinical research work are mainly in the treatment of new drugs, new methods of diagnosis, new technologies, new concepts and new methods of treatment. The experimental research is mainly to establish a variety of cancer-bearing models, to explore the mechanism and law of cancer onset, invasion and recurrence and metastasis, in order to find effective measures to regulate metastasis and recurrence and the experimental study on experimental screening of anticancer Chinese herbal medicines for cancer-bearing animals.

However, time to today, in the second decade of the 21st century, cancer is still rampant, the incidence rate is rising, and the mortality rate remains high.

I have been working in clinical oncology for 60 years. The more patients are treated, the more patients have. The incidence of cancer continues to rise. I am deeply aware that for cancer it should not only pay attention to treatment, but also attention should be paid to prevention in order to be at the source.

Therefore, I am deeply aware that the research work on cancer not only focuses on treatment, research on new drugs, new methods, new technologies, but also must focus on how to reduce the incidence of cancer.

How to stop the growing incidence of cancer continues to rise?

At present, the tumor hospital or oncology hospital model is fully focused on treatment, with emphasis on treatment and aiming at the middle and late patients. The curative effect is poor, the human resources are exhausted, and the incidence rate is not reduced, and the more patients are treated, the more patients come.

The status quo is:

The road that has passed in a century is to attention the treatment and ignore the prevention, or only to treat. For many years we have only been working or doing research on cancer treatment. However, work on cancer prevention has been done very little and almost nothing has been done. As a result, the incidence of cancer continues to rise.

Looking back or reflecting the old-fashioned cancer prevention and anti-cancer work, what research or work did we do in cancer prevention for a century? What has it been achieved?

Medical school textbook teaching content does not pay attention to cancer prevention knowledge.

The medical college model has not paid attention to the setting work of cancer prevention science.

Medical research projects in medical schools or hospitals have not paid attention to cancer prevention research projects.

The Journal of Oncology Medicine does not pay attention to cancer prevention work papers.

In short, cancer prevention has not been taken seriously, and prevention has not been taken seriously.

The prevention of the old-fashioned talks which is mainly based or the main focus is on failure to pay attention.

How to do? How to reduce the incidence of cancer? How to improve the cure rate of cancer? How to reduce cancer mortality? How to prolong the survival period? How to improve the quality of life?

It should be launched to overcome the general attack of cancer, prevention and treatment are equally important. The goal of conquering cancer should be:

Reduce morbidity, improve cure rate, reduce mortality, prolong survival, improve quality of life, and reduce complications.

At present, global hospitals and hospitals in China are all devoted to treatment, re-treatment and light prevention, or only treatment or cure.

XZ-C believes that this mode of hospitalization or cancer treatment is unlikely to overcome cancer and it is impossible to reduce the incidence.

Global hospitals and hospitals in China must carry out overall strategic reform of cancer treatment and swift from focusing on treatment into prevention and treatment at the same attention and at the same level.

Therefore, we propose to launch a general attack plan and design to overcome cancer. XZ-C (Xu Ze-China) (Xu Ze - China) proposed to launch a general attack, that is, the three stages of cancer prevention, cancer control and cancer treatment were carried out in full swing and simultaneously.

It is proposed the "Necessity and Feasibility Report for Overcoming the General Attack of Cancer Attack".

It is proposed "XZ-C Scientific Research Plan for Overcoming the General Attack of Cancer".

The focus of our research work in the fourth phase of cancer research in the past 28 years:

After 2011 -

Cancer research work, step by step in-depth

- Overall strategic reform with focusing on research goals and priorities for cancer treatment and turning focusing on treatment to focusing on prevention and treatment.

- We propose to launch a general attack to overcome cancer, which is to carry out the three-stage work of cancer prevention, cancer control and cancer treatment in the whole process of cancer occurrence and development, and carry out simultaneously.

That is:

Cancer prevention- before cancer formation

Cancer control - precancerous lesions with malignant tendencies

Treating cancer - has formed a cancerous foci or metastasis

- The goal of the total attack:

Reduce the incidence of cancer, reduce cancer mortality, improve cure rate, prolong survival, improve quality of life, and reduce complications.

- The need to launch a general attack on cancer

Why should I propose to launch a general attack?

Please look at the current situation:

—— The current situation of cancer incidence is that the more patients are treated and the more patients have, the average number of new cancer patients in China is 8,550, and 6 people per minute are diagnosed with cancer.

——The current status of cancer mortality is high, and it has been the leading cause of death in urban and rural areas in China. On average, 7,500 people die of cancer every day.

——The status quo of treatment, despite the application of traditional three major treatments for nearly a hundred years, thousands of cancer patients have been exposed to radiotherapy and chemotherapy, but what is the result?

Cancer is still the leading cause of death so far.

——The current status of the tumor hospital or oncology hospital model:

Attention to treatment and light prevention, or only cure, the more patients are treated and the more patients have.

- the feasibility of overcoming cancer and launching the general attack on cancer

Is there any scientific basis for launching a general attack on cancer?

Is there a medical basis?

Are there any favorable conditions for winning?

Although traditional therapies have failed to conquer cancer for nearly a century, the release and chemotherapy of traditional therapies cannot overcome cancer because it can only be relieved and cannot be cured.

It is feasible to propose a general attack, which is based on science and medicine.

Third

How to prevent cancer? I see three

How to overcome cancer, how to prevent cancer by I see three

(1) Why does it need to launch a general attack to conquer cancer?

(one)

Why is it proposed "to conquer cancer and it need to launch a general attack "?

1. Because the goal of conquering cancer should be:

(1) reduce the incidence of cance

It is to improve cancer cure rate, prolong patient survival and improve quality of life.

(2) reach

1/3 can prevent

1/3 can be cured

1/3 can prolong life through treatment

2, then, how can we reduce the incidence of cancer?

It should be prevention-oriented, control-oriented, and prevention-oriented.

But for decades, the road we have traveled is to attention treatment and ignore prevention or only to have treatment without prevention.

I have been working in clinical oncology surgery for 60 years. Looking back over the past few decades, the lesson of rethinking failure is that it can only be cured or treated without prevention, so the incidence of cancer is increasing, and the more patients are treated, the more patients have.

How to do?

It should be prevention-oriented, control-oriented, implement the prevention-oriented health work policy. Only to pay attention to preventing cancer can reduce the incidence of cancer. For cancer prevention and cancer control, how to prevent cancer? it should be the top priority or it should be the most important.

How can we implement and carry out the health work policy of prevention of cancer, cancer control, and prevention-oriented health work policy? How can we reform and correct the current mode of hospitalization, light defense, or treatment only ?

It is necessary to challenge the hospitality policy for cancer treatment, and reform can develop.

Professor Xu Ze proposed to launch the general attack, in fact, it is the prevention, control, and treatment at the same importance and it put cancer prevention and cancer control into the important parts. The essence is to implement and carry out the health work policy of "cancer prevention, anti-cancer" and "prevention-oriented".

Our medical predecessors and the world's medical sages put forward "cancer prevention, anti-cancer" and "prevention-oriented". This policy is very correct. Unfortunately, none of our medical juniors have paid much attention to it.

Especially our cancer researchers and health workers have not realized this. Over the past century, prevention has been neglected, cancer prevention has not been taken seriously, prevention has not been taken seriously, and cancer prevention has been neglected, leading to such a high incidence of cancer today. There are 8,550 new cancers in China every day, and 6 people are diagnosed with cancer every minute. It is so amazing data. It should be a national big event for the people's livelihood.

The task of health work should be "prevention of disease and treatment" and "prevention first". Health is to protect life and defend health. To launch the general attack, its essence is to put cancer prevention work at an important position, and to focus on reducing the incidence of cancer in order to prevent cancer and cancer.

Therefore, XZ-C proposed to overcome the general attack of cancer.

What is "launch the general attack" called?

The general attack is to prevent cancer, cancer control, and cancer treatment at the same time. The three carriages go hand in hand, in fact, it is the prevention, control, and treatment.

The essence of "Put cancer prevention and cancer control on important parts" is to implement the health work policy focusing on cancer prevention, cancer prevention and prevention.

It is a reform of the mode of running a hospital that emphasizes remediation or treatment with light prevention or only treatment without prevention, and only reform can develop.

So how to prevent cancer? What to prevent? How to prevent it? How to implement it?

In the search for the cause and condition of cancer, it is remarkable that it was found that more than 90% of cancers are caused by environmental factors. Therefore, XZ-C proposed to establish the cancer prevention research institute and the cancer prevention system project and conduct cancer prevention research, look for carcinogenic factors, detect the source of carcinogens or carcinogenic factors, and try to stop the damage caused by these carcinogenic factors, the Cancer Research Institute should conduct anti-cancer research. There is a lot of content that is urgently needed to be studied and they are very wide.

In order to track the source of carcinogens or carcinogenic factors, from what way or how should we proceed?
At present, with the improvement of people's living standards, while various high-tech products bring us a better life, it can also bring many negative effects. Various chemical, physical, and biological environmental carcinogens appear in large numbers. Various carcinogens enter our body or various carcinogenic factors affect our body to lead to an increasing incidence of cancer.
Because cancer is thought to be caused mainly by factors such as the environment, diet, and hobbies, therefore, people will attach great importance to carcinogenic factors in the environment and try to clear them.

In order to prevent cancer and control cancer, Professor Xu Ze proposed:

Cancer prevention should be carried out from clothing, food, shelter, and transportation. Cancer prevention should start from the big environment and small environment.

How to prevent cancer from clothing, food, shelter, and transportation?

First of all, you should master and understand the situation of carcinogens such as clothing, food, housing, and transportation and whether there will be a carcinogen or not?

It should be suitable for qualitative, quantitative, monitoring, then set the standard and set the bottom line to discuss. And it is to propose cancer prevention measures.

(2) The disaster of cancer covers the whole world

(two)

Cancer is a disaster for all mankind, and it must fight globally, and the global people struggle together

1. The disaster of cancer covers the whole world

The situation of worldwide cancer incidence

On the publication << the incidence of cancer in five continents>>, the 2002 volume of the publication was jointly published by the International Agency for Research on Cancer (IARC) and the International Association for Cancer Registration. It contains data on 50 cancers from 215 populations in 55 countries.

The IARC Special Report brings together findings from a cross-disciplinary panel of experts from different regions of the world on retrospective analysis of different potential carcinogenic risk factors. These panels evaluated a number of factors (including chemical factors, complex mixtures, occupational exposure factors, physical and biological factors, and lifestyle habits) to increase the risk of cancer risk.

Since 1971, the panel has evaluated more than 900 factors, of which nearly 400 have been identified as carcinogenic or potential carcinogenic factors. The full catalogue and classification of these factors is regularly updated and can be found on the website.

This catalogue is the scientific basis for public health, other disciplines, and national health authorities to take steps to avoid exposure to potential carcinogenic factors.

The situation of worldwide cancer incidence

There are great regional differences or variation widely around the world as well as some special organs about cancers morbidity and mortality rates. The WHO Cancer Mortality Database and the GLOBOCAN 2002 database provide data on the incidence, prevalence and mortality of 27 different cancers in each country in 2002.

In 2002, there were an estimated 10.9 million new cancer patients (53% male and 47% female), of which 5.1 million occurred in developed countries and 5.8 million occurred in less developed countries.

The number of cancer deaths was 6.7 million (57% male and 43% female), 2.7 million in developed countries and 4 million in less developed countries.

An estimated 24.5 million patients are still alive with various cancers (not including skin non-melanoma cancer within 5 years after diagnosis).

2. The situation of the mortality rate and current status of cancer patients worldwide

2017.2.5 Reference message

[Effie, Geneva, February 3rd]

The World Health Organization released data on the occasion of the "World Cancer Day" on February 4th.

At present, 8.8 million people die of cancer every year in the world, and among them the number of deaths from respiratory cancer is high, reaching 1.695 million per year.

The newly released data is based on 2015 statistics. The number of people dying from cancer each year has increased from an estimated 8.1 million in 2010 to 8.8 million.

The deadly cancers that are second only to respiratory cancer are liver cancer (788,000 deaths per year), colorectal cancer (774,000), stomach cancer (753,300) and breast cancer (571,000).

Cancers such as esophageal cancer (415,000), pancreatic cancer (358,000), prostate cancer (334,800), and lymphoma (334,300) also have high mortality rates worldwide.

In terms of gender, there are nearly 5 million male deaths among 8.8 million cancer deaths. For men, the types of cancer with high mortality rate are respiratory cancer and liver cancer.

For women, cancers with high mortality rate are breast cancer and respiratory cancer.

In terms of regional distribution, the majority or the most of cancer cases are in the western Pacific, where respiratory cancer and liver cancer account for a high proportion.

The second only to the Western Pacific is Southeast Asia, where respiratory cancer, oral cancer and throat cancer account for a high proportion.

In Europe, deadly cancer is also a respiratory cancer, followed by colorectal cancer.

The disaster of cancer covers the whole world. People all over the world are eager to hope that one day they will be able to overcome cancer. It is hoped that countries, governments, experts, scholars, and scientists will find out cancer prevention measures to keep people away from cancer.

3. Currently, the status quo of 5-year survival rate of cancer globally

Today, the current state of the global cancer 5-year survival rate is still at a lower level

It can be said that there are more and more methods and means available to clinicians today in the clinical diagnosis and treatment of tumors. But we have to face up to reality, numerous analyses of clinical epidemiology suggest that the maturity and development of diagnostic capabilities and means does not seem to be fully synchronized with the overall therapeutic effect of the tumor. **According to the data distributed by The American Cancer Society (pictured), in the past ten years, the level of diagnosis and treatment of various malignant tumors has been greatly improved compared with the past, but its 5-year survival rate is still lingering at a lower level.** For example, the 5-year survival rate of global colon cancer in 2004 was 62%. Although the diagnostic techniques and surgical treatment of colon cancer have made great progress, but currently only increased to 65%, no breakthroughs have been made. The etiology, epidemiological studies and various treatment techniques of liver cancer have been greatly improved.

However, the current 5-year survival rate is only 18%, which is only 11 percentage points higher than 10 years ago. How to improve the prognosis of patients is still a problem that plagues hepatobiliary surgeons. The mortality rate of gastric cancer has been high. Although the level of surgical technology has been continuously improved, the 5-year survival rate of gastric cancer has only increased from 23% 10 years ago to 29%. In addition, the 5-year survival rate of pancreatic cancer is not much changed from 10 years ago, and it is lingering up and down at 5%; the 5-year survival rate of esophageal cancer has been maintained at 14%; the 5-year survival rate for breast cancer has dropped from 87% 10 years ago to 79% today. Cervical cancer has dropped from 71% to 69%. The 5-year survival rate for lung cancer has also dropped from 15% to the current 14%.

(3) XZ-C proposed to establish cancer prevention research institute and cancer prevention system project

XZ-C proposes that in order to overcome cancer and to launch the general attack on cancer, it is necessary to establish advice and suggestions for the Cancer Research Institute and the cancer prevention system project.

Conducting cancer research, looking for carcinogenic factors, detecting the source of carcinogens or carcinogenic factors, and try to stop the damage caused by these carcinogenic factors; the Cancer Research Institute should conduct anti-cancer research; the content which needs to do the research urgent is many and wide.

Track the source of carcinogens or carcinogenic factors.

While Human beings are looking for the cause and condition of cancer,

Prominently, it was found that more than 90% of cancers are caused by environmental factors.

How is it to implement the creation of this cancer prevention research institute?

Professor Xu Ze (XZ-C) proposed the general design of cancer prevention and proposed cancer prevention system engineering:

The way in which so many carcinogens or carcinogenic factors should be studied

Study these sources of pollution,

Try to stop at the source

Study these carcinogenic mechanisms and their carcinogenic effects

Study how to reduce or prevent these carcinogens

Because cancer patients cover the whole world, and the pollution of industrial and agricultural wastewater, waste residue and waste gas also cover the whole world, therefore, it is imperative that the global effort be made to overcome cancer and to launch the general attack on cancer.

(4) Advocating scientific research ethics, medicine is benevolence, and setting up ethics is the first

Professor Xu Ze suggested:

1. All countries, provinces and states should establish anti-cancer research institutes (or institutions), carry out cancer prevention system projects, and carry out cancer prevention work for their own country, province and city.

2. Countries establish cancer prevention regulations and carry out comprehensively (some should be legislated)

3. I will use this project to recommend the World Health Organization to hold the cancer prevention campaign, with the goal of reducing the incidence of cancer.

Conquering cancer is the frontier of science, a worldwide problem, and cancer is a human disaster and covering the globe, people all over the world are eager to hope that one day they will be able to conquer cancer and benefit humanity.

4. **To advocate scientific research ethics; medicine is benevolence; the ethics is set up first**

Research ethics: products should have ethical standards

Standard: it should be based on the standard of not damaging to human health

Basic ethics: All products should be harmless to people and do not harm people's health, especially for children.

(To be beautiful and clear mountain and transparent water and living environment and surviving environment with birds and flowers)

5. The health administrative department shall protect life and protect health, and shall fugle, lead, support, and guide anti-cancer measures, cancer prevention projects, cancer prevention tests, and cancer prevention monitoring.

Cancer is a disaster for all mankind. It must fight with the world and the people of the world will work together. Human beings should not sit still, doctors should not do nothing, and the health administration should not do nothing. It should fugle and lead the cancer prevention research series project, move together, work together, complement each other, lead and guide to overcome cancer and launch a general attack.

Fourth

How to prevent cancer? I see four

How to overcome cancer? In order to overcome cancer, we must create << The Research Institute of an innovative environmental protection and cancer prevention research>>.

--------it is one of the science cities to overcome cancer.

(1) Why the research institute of the innovative environmental protection and cancer prevention should be built?

Why should we create an innovative environmental protection and cancer prevention research institute? It is because: the current cancer incidence is on the rise, 90% of which is related to the environment.

The occurrence of cancer is closely related to people's clothing, food, housing, travel and living habits.

The current environmental pollution is serious and the ecosystem is degraded, which may be related to the cancer incidence rate.

After 28 years of retrospective and reflection on the experimental research and clinical work of cancer research work, we deeply understand that for cancer it should not only pay attention to treatment, but also pay attention to prevention, so as to stop cancer at the source. It must be prevention and treatment, and the way out to fight cancer is prevention and prevention is the main factor.

So how to prevent it ? What to prevent? It is necessary to measure, characterize, locate, and quantify various environmental carcinogens and try to remove them.

Therefore, it is necessary to establish cancer prevention research institute, which should conduct cancer prevention research from clothing, food, housing, and transportation, and carry out microscopic and ultra-microscopic anti-cancer research from the big environment and small environment.

How to conduct cancer prevention research from clothing, food, housing and transportation? First of all, you should master the situation of clothing, food, shelter, and other carcinogens, whether it contains carcinogens or not?

It should be qualitative and quantitative monitoring, and then set standards and set the bottom line, in order to discuss and propose prevention and control measures.

(2) How to create research institute of the innovative environmental protection and cancer prevention?

How to create the "Cancer Research Institute with Innovative Environmental Protection and cancer prevention "?

Cancer prevention research is a major event. At present, there is no cancer prevention research institute in the world. We will apply to create "the world's first environmentally friendly cancer prevention Research Institute" to monitor macro, micro, ultra-micro environmental carcinogens, analysis, implementation of cancer prevention systems engineering in the Science City of conquering Cancer".

How to overcome cancer? In order to overcome cancer, it is necessary to launch a general attack. The general attack is to comprehensively carry out the three stages of cancer prevention, cancer control, and cancer treatment in the whole process of cancer occurrence and development, and simultaneously carry out prevention, control, and treatment at the same time and at the same level.

With the improvement of people's living standards, various high-tech products bring us a better life, but also bring many negative effects. Various chemical, physical, and biological environmental carcinogens appear in large numbers. Various carcinogens enter our human body or various carcinogenic factors affect our human body, leading to an increasing incidence of cancer.

Please look at the current situation:

The current state of cancer incidence is that the more patients are treated and the more patients have. The current incidence of cancer in China is 3.12 million new cases of cancer each year. On average, there are 8550 new cancer patients per day. Six people were diagnosed with cancer every minute in the country.

Now XZ-C proposes to the scientific research plan for overcoming cancer and launch the general attack of cancer; the prevention, control, and treatment are equally important, and the three carriages go hand in hand.

So how to prevent it? How to control? What to prevent? What to control? How much? How much is controlled?

The target or "target" of the prevention or control must be clear; qualitative, quantitative, and localization must be measured for various environmental carcinogens.

Since cancer is thought to be caused mainly by factors such as the environment, diet, and hobbies, people will attach great importance to carcinogenic factors in the environment and strive to remove them.

(3) Professor Xu Ze proposed: cancer prevention should be carried out from clothing, food, shelter and transportation, and cancer prevention should be carried out from the big environment and small environment

In order to prevent cancer and control cancer, Professor Xu Ze proposed:

(1) Cancer prevention should be carried out from clothing, food, shelter, and transportation, and cancer prevention should be carried out from a large environment or a small environment.

(2) The following anti-cancer research groups should be formed, and the graduate students of each school should be invited to complete and complete this scientific research work.

Professor Xu Ze, as the chief designer, proposes the following research projects and topics. To overcome cancer, the following research work must be carried out:

(1) Know what needs to be prevented? What needs to be controlled? How to prevent? How to control?

It must be qualitative, quantitative, and location monitoring, have clear and specific data. It is necessary to master the first-hand information in order to carry out cancer prevention work scientifically and accurately, and must pay attention to the accumulation of original materials as a scientific data and experimental basis for accurate cancer prevention.

(2) How to achieve this plan? How to carry out this scientific research work?

It can be included in the training of graduate students and it can be selected by doctoral students and master students. It can not only train postgraduate for field research, but also receive monitoring and analysis of the qualitative and quantitative of the components or ingredients for carcinogen or cancer prevention things, to further propose prevention and control measures and methods.

Method:

Graduate students from various universities set up tasks, have purpose, have task arrangement

(My graduate student is like this, The general subject of the tutor is like a table banquet. Each graduate student is a small topic. As stir-fried dishes, doctoral students fry a large plate and master students fry a small plate). This gives full play to the role of graduate students. It can also cultivate graduate students' scientific thinking, scientific practice ability, produce papers, produce talents, and produce results.

It must emphasize graduate research papers, and it is not written with a pen, but it is made by scientific research. We must pay attention to the original materials, attach importance to scientific and technological innovation, and attach importance to the advanced, innovative and practical. We must pay attention to scientific research and seek truth from facts.

Create the research institute of the environmental protection and cancer prevention and carry out cancer prevention system engineering

How to prevent cancer from clothing, food, shelter, and transportation?

First of all, you should master and understand the situation of carcinogens such as clothing, food, housing, and transportation.

Whether it contains carcinogens, qualitative and quantitative monitoring, then set standards, set the bottom line, then it can be discussed to propose prevention and control measures.

It is planned to establish the following research groups:

(1) [clothing]

The research group of Carcinogen monitoring, prevention and control for clothes, cosmetics, etc.

Purpose:

Method:

Technology:

Equipment conditions:

Personnel:

Expected results and achievements :

With or without carcinogens, qualitative, quantitative, red bottom line, microscopic, ultra-microscopic monitoring

Analysis and conclusion:

proposing for prevention and control measures, or further experimenting the animal models

Graduate student (master and Ph.D)

resulting in:

(2) [Food]

Food Carcinogen Monitoring, Prevention and Control Research Group → Institute

Pickled products:

Carcinogen content monitoring and qualitative and quantitative microscopic research, such as kimchi, grilled vegetables, dried salted fish, sausage, mustard, bacon, fermented bean curd, pickles, canned fish, etc.

Frying method:

... and other carcinogen content monitoring, qualitative and quantitative microscopic research

Fried method:

... and other carcinogen content monitoring, qualitative and quantitative microscopic research

Smoke method:

... and other carcinogen content monitoring, qualitative and quantitative microscopic research

Cooking method:

... and other carcinogen content monitoring, qualitative and quantitative microscopic research

Steaming method:

... and other carcinogen content monitoring, qualitative and quantitative microscopic research

Fume stove:

... and other carcinogen content monitoring, qualitative and quantitative microscopic research

Leftovers:

... and other carcinogen content monitoring, qualitative and quantitative microscopic research

Leftovers overnight:

... and other carcinogen content monitoring, qualitative and quantitative microscopic research

grain:

... and other carcinogen content monitoring, qualitative and quantitative microscopic research

oil:

... and other carcinogen content monitoring, qualitative and quantitative microscopic research

vegetables:

... and other carcinogen content monitoring, qualitative and quantitative microscopic research

meat:

... and other carcinogen content monitoring, qualitative and quantitative microscopic research

Fish:

... and other carcinogen content monitoring, qualitative and quantitative microscopic research

Various foods (packaged) are sold by supermarkets.

(3) [Living]:

Housing, decoration (painting, paint enamel) materials, furniture ······

Carcinogen Monitoring, Prevention and Control Research Group

Determination of materials, air, micro, ultra-microscopic carcinogens

Whether it exceeds the standard (for several large advertising companies...)

Trace element determination and monitoring

(4) [Travelling]:

Automotive Exhaust, Carbide Monitoring, Prevention and Control Research Group

Cars, trains, etc., air

Train:

Aircraft:

Battery car

(5) Water, pollution (waste water, air in each plant) carcinogen monitoring, prevention, control, research group

(6) Fertilizer, pesticide, soil grain, genetically modified food, whether there is carcinogen monitoring, prevention, control, research group

(7) Monitoring, prevention, control, research group on whether computers or mobile phones have carcinogenic or damaging effects

(8) Air, air conditioner, range hood, radiation, radiation, nuclear radiation measurement, carcinogen monitoring, prevention, control, research group

(9) Chinese food and western food are all qualitatively and quantitatively monitored for carcinogenicity, qualitative, quantitative, and standard

·The goal of the study:

to detect whether there are carcinogens and their content, qualitative, quantitative, standard

·Methods:

Layout of doctoral and master's programs, projects

Initial screening, preliminary research, to find problems → ask questions → study problems → solve problems

·Participants:

chefs, dieticians, tutors, postgraduate colleges, canteens, hotels, restaurants, snacks, hot dry noodles, flour

Graduate students go to the site to conduct research, experiment, practice and carry out scientific research work.

Tutor - Graduate - Nutritional Expert Trinity Monitoring, Research, Analysis

·The overall layout of the project, the purpose, the request

It can be a college which is responsible for one problem.

· Layout 100 graduate students, ie 100 papers, preliminary on the carcinogen composition, quantitative, qualitative monitoring, analysis

Funding subsidies:

·It will strive for support and guidance from the Education Department, the Science and Technology Department, the Eco-Environment Department, and the Health and Health Commission.

· It will strive for support, guidance, and leadership from various colleges, and you will probably acquire a large number of scientific research results in epidemiology, nutrition, preventive medicine, public health, and environmental science, and grasp first-hand information for cancer prevention and cancer control.

"Three Early" Study

The research of the early diagnosis technology, early diagnosis reagent to search for early diagnosis methods and reagents:

1. Monitor changes in trace elements:

Normal person: 500 cases

Precancerous lesions: 500 cases

Various cancer people: 500 cases

Various patients: 500 cases

Specimen cut by various tumors: 500 cases

Create the research institute of the environmental protection and cancer prevention and carry out cancer prevention system engineering

Specimens: blood, urine, saliva, feces, sputum

```
        Inflammatory      neoplasia
    ─────────────────┼─────────────────
                     │
              Boundary monitoring
          Before treatment: after treatment
```

2. Immune monitoring

Normal person: 500 cases

Precancerous lesions: 500 cases

Various cancer people: 500 cases

Various patients: 500 cases

Various cancer specimens: 500 cases

Various cancers before surgery: 500 cases

Postoperative: 500 cases

Before chemotherapy: 500 cases

After chemotherapy: 500 cases

1 time

2 times

3 times

4 times

Before radiotherapy: 500 cases

After radiotherapy: 500 cases

3. Monitoring of endocrine hormones

Monitoring of the relationship between ovarian function and milk Ca: 500 cases

Monitoring the relationship between ovarian function and cervical Ca and ovarian cancer Find the baseline and baseline limits and monitoring: 500 cases

4. Correlation analysis of hemorheology monitoring and metastasis: 500 cases

Correlation analysis of blood coagulability monitoring and metastasis: 500 cases

Correlation analysis between microcirculation monitoring and micro-cancer: 500 cases

5. Correlation analysis between genetic testing and clinical manifestations (symptoms and signs)

Analysis of genetic detection and pathophysiology, metabolic function and compensatory function

Is genetic testing a cause or a consequence?

Combined analysis and argumentation

6. Study on the combination of tumor markers with clinical analysis and grading

7. CEA↑ AFP↑ PSA↑

Does it represent Ca Cell? Can killing Ca Cell be effective? How to deal with it?

8. Early diagnosis, only qualitative, not positioned, how to deal with? What kind of medicine is used?

Fifth

XZ-C proposes to create the "the Research Institute of the Innovative Environmental Protection and Cancer Prevention" and carry out cancer prevention system engineering

Scientific research plan
Original innovation
Secret level: Class A

XZ-C proposes to create the "Innovative Environmental Protection and Cancer Research Institute" and carry out anti-cancer system engineering.

XZ-C proposes: Twilight anti-cancer plan A, B, D

Under the guidance of Xi Jinping's new era of socialism with Chinese characteristics, we should work hard to open up new prospects for scientific research in the new era. Research work to overcome cancer should go forward. During this new era, new journey, new action, new weather, it is to be a courageous person in the new era.

Under the guidance of Xi Jinping's new era of socialism with Chinese characteristics, it is to strive to take the road of self-innovation with Chinese characteristics and to adhere to the road of independent innovation of the combination of Chinese and Western medicine with "Chinese-style anti-cancer". China will contribute more Chinese wisdom, China programs, and Chinese power to the world so that the sun of the humanity's destiny will shine in the world. Let the sun of the human destiny share the sun.

How to overcome cancer? How to prevent cancer?

XZ-C proposes: Create "Cancer Research Institute of Innovative Environmental Protection" and carry out cancer prevention system engineering

How to overcome cancer? How to prevent cancer?

XZ-C proposes to create the "Cancer Research Institute of Innovative Environmental Protection" and carry out cancer prevention system engineering

XZ-C proposes:

Dawning A type cancer prevention plan

Dawning B type cancer prevention plan

Dawning D-type cancer prevention plan

Macro, micro, ultra-micro

Combine with the three major challenges, ride research, fouling prevention, pollution control, cancer prevention, anti-cancer

1. **XZ-C proposed that in order to overcome cancer and to launch the general attack on cancer, it must establish the Cancer Research Institute and the cancer prevention system project. This is the first time internationally proposed.**

Conduct cancer prevention research, find cancer-causing factors, detect the source of carcinogens or carcinogenic factors, and try to stop the human body damage caused by these carcinogenic factors. The Cancer Research Institute should conduct cancer prevention research.

There is a lot of very wide content that is urgently needed to be studied.

Track the source of carcinogens or carcinogenic factors.

While human beings are looking for the cause and condition of cancer, the most prominent is the discovery that more than 90% of cancers are caused by environmental factors.

(1) Relationship between air pollution and cancer

Humans have developed tens of millions of tons of coal, oil and natural gas as fuel and energy. In the production and life processes such as thermal power generation, smelting steel, automobiles, airplanes, and household fuels, **a large amount of tar, bituminous coal, dust and other harmful substances are discharged into the atmosphere around the clock, causing air pollution.**

Air pollution can cause many diseases, especially respiratory diseases, the most serious is lung cancer.

(2) Water pollution and cancer

The pollution of water quality is mainly caused by industrial and agricultural production and urban sewage. There are many types of pollutants in water. **Insecticides and pesticides are one of the important pollutants in water. Surfactants in neutral detergents also have cancer-promoting effects.**

(3) Soil pollution and cancer

A large amount of industrial waste water residue and pesticides and fertilizers are injected into the soil, **which deteriorates soil quality and accumulates poisons, posing a threat to human health and a carcinogenic factor.**

(4) Chemistry and cancer

(5) Physical factors and cancer

(6) Biological factors and cancer

(7) Diet and cancer

(8) Lifestyle and cancer

(9) clothing, food, housing, transportation, house decoration, etc. and cancer

The working way of so many carcinogens or carcinogenic factors should be studied.

Study these sources of pollution and try to stop at the source

Study these carcinogenic mechanisms and their carcinogenic effects

Study how to reduce or prevent these carcinogens

2. It is proposed for the first time in the world:

XZ-C proposes Dawning Anti-cancer Program A, B, D for anti-fouling, pollution control, anti-cancer, anti-cancer

Dawning Type A Plan: Goal: Prevent Air Pollution

Dawning B-type plan: Goal: Prevent water pollution

Dawning D-type plan: goal: to prevent soil pollution

How to overcome cancer? How to prevent cancer? I see:

Professor Xu Ze proposed that the "Innovative Environmental Protection and Cancer Research Institute" should be established and the cancer prevention system project should be carried out.

Where is the target or "target" of cancer prevention? How to prevent?

The more cancer patients are treated more and more, the incidence is rising, and 90% of them are related or closely related to environmental carcinogenic factors. **Therefore, the target or "target" of cancer prevention should be to study, explore and take scientific prevention and treatment measures against the carcinogenic factors (external environment, internal environment) of the environment.**

XZ-C proposes cancer prevention general design and cancer prevention system engineering:

Since the disaster of cancer covers the whole world, industrial and agricultural waste gas, waste water and waste residue also cover the whole world. Therefore, it is necessary to establish the "Cancer Research Institute with Innovative Environmental Protection" and carry out cancer prevention system engineering.

It is necessary to prevent and control the three major pollutions, and it is advisable to study the relationship between the environment and cancer.

Such as ensuring the relationship between environmental pollution and cancer, there are many examples in history, especially air pollution, water pollution, and soil pollution. In particular, the environmental pollution has a serious impact on human carcinogenesis.

(1) Air pollution in environmental pollution and cancer:

Human beings cannot be separated from air every minute of their lives, that means that every minute of human life is inseparable from the air Air pollution can cause many respiratory diseases, of which lung cancer is severe or among them, lung cancer is serious.

(2) Water pollution in environmental pollution and cancer:

Human beings can't live without water every time they are in production activities and life. Water pollution is mainly caused by industrial and agricultural production and urban sewage.

In China, industrial pollution has intensified due to the rapid development of township and village enterprises. Water pollution is associated with high incidence of lung cancer and is associated with gastric cancer, intestinal cancer, and esophageal cancer. Drinking unqualified water that does not meet the standard can induce or promote cancer.

(3) Soil pollution in environmental pollution and cancer:

Fertilizers, pesticides and insecticides in agricultural production can lead to soil water quality, serious soil pollution, agricultural workers exposure to a variety of pesticides, herbicides and fertilizers, some of which are known as human carcinogens.

Fouling prevention and pollution control is actually cancer prevention and cancer control. It can effectively prevent the effects of first-class cancer prevention. It must prevent and control the three major pollutions, pollution prevention, pollution control, and overcome difficulties. It can certainly achieve the benefits of cancer prevention and cancer control, reduce the incidence of cancer.

3. XZ-C proposed and formulated four Dawning Cancer Prevention Programs, which was first proposed internationally.

The Cancer Research Institute will carry out cancer prevention system engineering, conduct microscopic, ultra-micro, high-tech research, monitor and analyze carcinogenic factors, and try to remove, we have developed four Dawning Cancer Prevention Programs:

1). Dawn A type plan:

aims:

Try microscopic study of air pollution on carcinogenic factors environmental research, and try to remove in order toprevent lung cancer caused by air pollution.

Why is the cancer prevention system project the first to solve air pollution? It is because the current global respiratory cancer has been the highest incidence rate,

1.295 million / 8.18 million, both male and female are the first. Therefore, how to solve the problem of preventing lung cancer is a top priority.

Ways and methods:

Through microscopic, ultra-micro, high-tech monitoring and analysis of carcinogenic factors, try to detect, monitor, and try to remove it.

2). Dawn B plan

Aims:

Try to study the microscopic study of the carcinogenic factors of water pollution on the environment, and try to remove cancers such as liver cancer, stomach cancer, and intestinal cancer caused by waterproof pollution.

Why does wawe must pay attention to water pollution and cancer?

Why do it must pay attention to that water pollution causes cancer at present?

It is because the mother rivers of the whole country and the whole world are discharged by industrial and agricultural sewage and urban sewage. River water is in pollution, carcinogens increased significantly. Professor Xu Ze (XZ-C) suggested that efforts should be made to save the mother river of the whole country and the world from being seriously polluted.

Ways and methods:

"target"

In order to solve the pollution of industrial and agricultural sewage, the first should try to reduce fertilizer.

In order to solve urban and rural drinking water, it must be purified and qualified.

To resolve drinking water qualified and to drink standard water

3). Dawn C plan

Already mentioned above

4). Dawn D plan

Aims or objectives:

Try to research the microscopic study of the carcinogenic factors of soil pollution on the environment

Try to solve the problem of chemical fertilizers, pesticides, genetic modification and the occurrence of cancer

Try to detect the presence or absence of carcinogenic factors from clothing, food, housing, and samples, and take samples of the amount of carcinogens from microscopic monitoring.

The ways and methods:

Conduct microscopic detection and monitoring of cancer prevention, and put forward ethical standards for cancer prevention.

Through the above-mentioned Dawning A, B, and D plans, fouling prevention and pollution control of the atmosphere, water, and soil are actually a first-level cancer prevention, which can reduce the incidence of cancer. It can reach the ecological environment of green hills, green waters, mountains and rivers, birds and flowers, and human living environment.

Because cancer patients cover the whole world, the pollution of industrial and agricultural wastewater, waste residue and waste gas also covers the whole world. Therefore, it is imperative that the global effort be made to overcome conquer and to launch the general attack on cancer.

Professor Xu Ze suggested:

1). All countries, provinces and states should establish cancer prevention research institutes (or institutions), carry out cancer prevention system projects, and carry out cancer prevention work for their own country, province and city.

2). Countries establish cancer prevention regulations and carry out comprehensively (some should be legislated)

3). I will use this project to recommend the World Health Organization to hold cancer prevention campaign, with the goal of reducing the incidence of cancer. Conquering cancer is the frontier of science, a worldwide problem, cancer is a human disaster, covering the global, people all over the world are eager to hope that one day they will be able to conquer cancer and benefit humanity. One day it can overcome cancer and benefit mankind.

Six

Conduct scientific research on cancer control and prevention and formulate cancer control plans and measures

Conduct scientific research on cancer control and prevention

----- Formulating plans and measures for cancer control

Carry on the medical science research on cancer control and prevention, Make the planning and measures for cancer control

(1) Relationship between environmental pollution and cancer

(2) Relationship between lifestyle and cancer

(3) Relationship between diet and cancer

(4) Personal Prevention of Cancer

(5) Self-early discovery of cancer

(6) Prospects for cancer prevention research in the 21st century

Foreword

Why does it need to "develop medical science research on cancer control and prevention"?

Why does it need to "Develop the planning and measures for cancer control"?

At present, our city is standing at a new development starting point.

In-depth implementation of the strategy is for the rise of the central region. The construction of a "two-oriented society" has created a major opportunity for the development of Wuhan. Under this great situation and great opportunities, it also created a good opportunity for research work on cancer prevention and cancer prevention. It is conducive to scientific research on cancer prevention and cancer control and improve people's awareness of cancer prevention. The purpose is for the health of the people, keep away from cancer and reduce the incidence of cancer in our province and city.

Current cancer trends and faced challenges is that more experts, scholars and people with lofty ideals are needed to conduct medical scientific research on cancer prevention and control.

1. Cancer has become a major public health problem worldwide. Compared with other chronic diseases, cancer prevention and control will face greater challenges: the occurrence of cancer is related to environmental pollution, lifestyle, diet, life behavior, and psychosocial factors.

2. According to the International Cancer Research Center report:

The number of cancers is increasing at an average annual rate of 3.5%.

The number of morbidity and deaths increased by 24.7% and 19.2%, respectively, compared with 10 years ago.

In the past 30 years, the mortality rate of cancer in China has been on the rise. It has become the first cause of death for urban and rural residents. On average, one out of every four deaths has died of cancer:

The primary cause of death in urban and rural residents in China in 2006 was cancer.

In 2008 compared with 2006, the proportion of cancer deaths increased by nearly 2-fold.

China has 160 million people with cancer each year, 1.3 million people die from cancer each year, and an annual rate of 3% annually. Preventing cancer, changing bad lifestyles, and developing a healthy lifestyle are imminent.

3. Cancer not only poses a serious threat to human health, but also an important factor in the rapid rise of medical expenses:

The direct cost of cancer treatment in China is nearly 100 billion yuan per year, which is a huge economic burden for patients and society as a whole.

4. Although countries have invested heavily in the treatment of cancer patients, the 5-year survival rate of some common cancers has not improved significantly in the past 20 years. Despite nearly three hundred years of traditional treatment, cancer is still the leading cause of death for urban and rural residents in China. How to do? How should the road go? It should be analyzed, reflected, and studied.

5. For malignant tumors, the way to fight cancer is prevention. The United Nations Health Organization proposes that one-third of cancers can be prevented.

It has become the consensus of cancer researchers to carry out active and effective early warning, early diagnosis and intervention research to reduce the incidence of cancer and improve the cure rate.

Honorary President and Professor of Surgery, Wuhan Anticancer Research Society

In China. Hubei, Wuhan

April 2019

Conduct research on cancer control and prevention and develop cancer control plans and measures

(1) Relationship between environmental pollution and cancer

In today's prosperous times, people's living standards continue to improve, and various high-tech products have brought us a better life, but also brought a variety of chemical, physical, and biological environmental carcinogens. Various carcinogens enter our body or various carcinogenic factors affect our body. People seem to be shrouded in the oceans of environmentally harmful carcinogens.

While some people talk about cancer, their skin color changes, and it seems that the grass are all soldiers; Others are insensitive and do whatever they do in life.

Cancer is not terrible. What is terrible is that we don't have simple basic knowledge about cancer prevention. Most cancers can be prevented.

Why do we link energy conservation and environmental protection with the research of cancer prevention and cancer control ?

What is energy saving? What is emission reduction? What is the environment? What is environmentally friendly type?

First, let talk about what the environment is ?

The environment in which humans live includes: natural and social environment. What is the natural environment? That is to surround the various natural factors around people. For example, everyone should breathe air, water and food. These common physical environments are called the big environment.

Everyone must engage in certain work and adopt a certain lifestyle, such as occupation, living habits and hobbies, to form a living environment called a small environment.

Whether it is a large environment or a small environment, it is the external environment on which human beings depend for survival and activity.

The physiological condition of the human body is called the internal environment.

The external environment substances have a close relationship with the internal environment through the ingestion, digestion, absorption, metabolism and excretion of the organism, which has a huge impact on the human body.

How to prove the relationship between environmental pollution and cancer?

There are many examples in history:

Relationship between environment and cancer

In the process of searching for the cause and condition of cancer, human beings have carried out extensive exploration and accumulated rich knowledge. More than 90% of cancers were found to be caused by environmental factors or closely related.

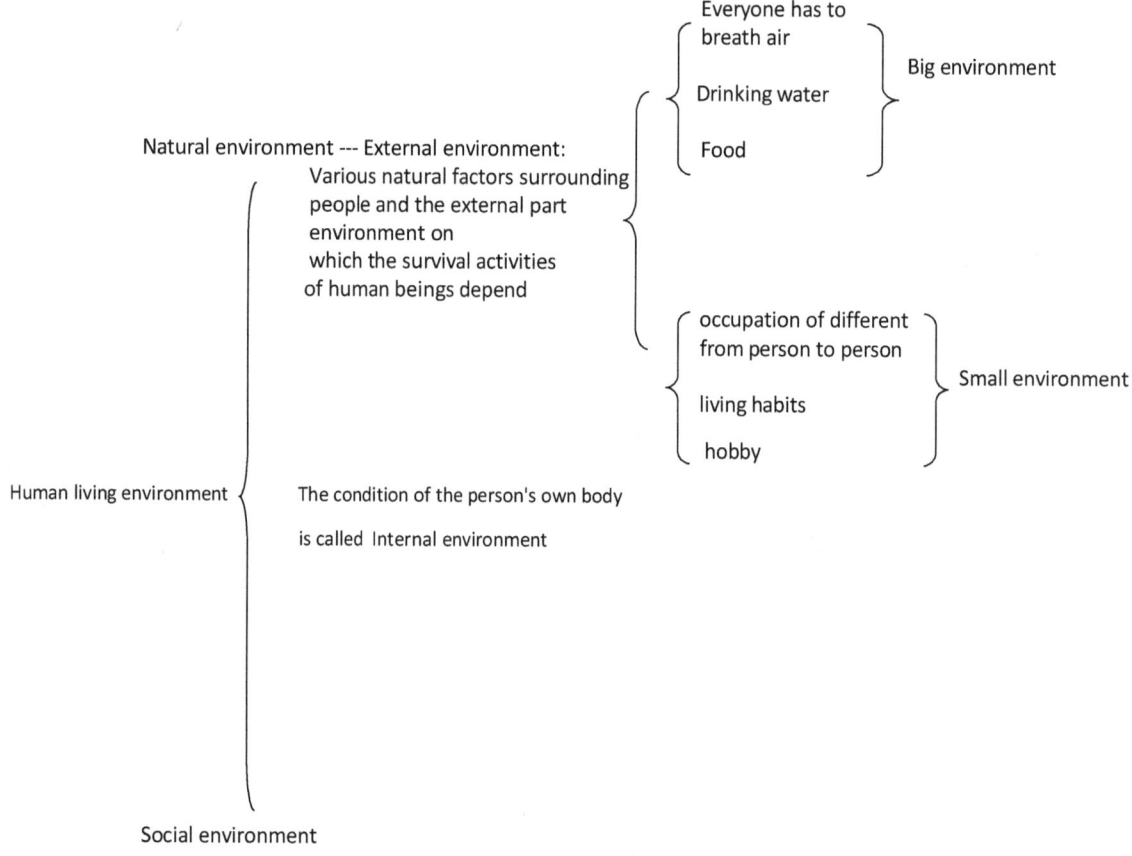

The relation of environmental pollution and cancer

There are the historical examples:

1). In 1775, Dr. Port of England confirmed that there were many scrotal skin cancers among workers who cleaned the chimney. The main reason is the long-term exposure to tobacco tar. This is the first historical example of linking cancer to environmental factors.

2). After 100 years, German doctor Volkman also realized that the high incidence of skin cancer among workers may be related to exposure to coal tar.

3). Sun exposure was found to be associated with skin cancer in 1907, which is the first reported epidemiological studies of sunlight and skin cancer. The researchers observed early on that the crew were exposed to solar radiation and caused chronic skin disease, which is a very common phenomenon. Later, animal models confirmed that daylight and ultraviolet light can cause skin cancer.

4). An animal model of the first chemical agent-induced tumor was established in 1915. Repeated application of tar can cause skin cancer in rabbits. This study added experimental evidence for the establishment of a chemical carcinogenic theory based on the scrotal cancer of chimney cleaners in 1775. Later, the active ingredient, coal tar, was confirmed and isolated.

5). In the 20th century it was confirmed that there is high incidence of bladder cancer in workers producing methylnaphthylamine, ethylnaphthylamine and benzidine dyes and almost all engaged workers who have passed this occupation have developed bladder cancer or almost all workers who had such occupations subsequently developed bladder cancer.

6). In 1930, the first chemical carcinogen, benzo(a)pyrene, was separated from coal tar. Known carcinogenic environmental substances, coal tar, are separated into different components, and the carcinogenic effects of these chemical components are clarified by animal model experiments.

7). The 1938 study found that the chemical carcinogenic process is divided into two distinct phases, the stimulating phase and the priming phase. Non-specific stimuli promote tumorigenesis after low-dose carcinogens, such as tar or nipple on the ears. Rhonavirus.

8) In 1938 the study found that the chemical carcinogenesis process is divided into two different stages: initiation phase and triggering phase. Non-specific stimuli promote tumorigenesis after challenge with low doses of carcinogens, such as tar or papilloma virus on the ears.

9) In 1940, researchers found that limiting calories reduced the incidence of murine tumors, proving that caloric intake can contribute to several tumors such as breast cancer, liver cancer and skin cancer induced by benzopyrene. Until today's obesity is prevalent in the world, this work has once again received attention.

10). Epidemiological studies in 1950 found that smoking was associated with lung cancer. Retrospective analysis of lung cancer patients with smoking habits has shown that smoking is associated with lung cancer.

Later studies in male doctors showed that smoking has a significant relationship with lung cancer mortality. Smoking has now proven to be a dangerous cause for many cancers, it can increase the mortality rate of cancer by about 30%.

11). Food additives banned by the Food Additive Improvement Agency in 1958 induced the development of cancer in humans or animals.

12). In 1964, American surgeon Luther LTerry suggested that smoking is associated with lung cancer.

13). Vinyl chloride is the main raw material for the plastics industry. It was not until 1974 that scientists discovered that this chemical is a potentially potent carcinogen that can cause liver cancer.

Epidemiological investigations in recent decades have found that many occupational workers are exposed to carcinogens in the production environment, and the incidence of cancer in some areas is greatly increased. When these occupational exposures are eliminated or avoided, the onset of these cancers can be gradually reduced or even disappeared. It shows that environmental factors play a major role in the process of tumorigenesis.

The long-term effects of various environmental factors other than the human body are the main causes of most cancers. Therefore, we should minimize the impact of these environmental, living and behavioral factors on the human body and stay away from cancer.

Let's talk about the serious effects of environmental pollution such as air pollution, water pollution and soil pollution on human carcinogenesis:

1. Air pollution in environmental pollution and cancer

(1) Sources of air pollution

Humans have developed tons of tons of coal, oil and natural gas as fuel and energy. In the production and life processes such as thermal power generation, smelting steel, automobiles and airplanes, as well as domestic living fuels, a large amount of harmful gases such as coal tar, soot and dust are discharged into the atmosphere around the clock.

It is estimated that more than 80% of the environmental pollutants in the atmosphere come from the combustion process of fuel. Because of these increasing emissions, these large amounts of poison gas are concentrated in the city.

Under the action of light energy, pollutants in the air will also undergo complex photochemical reactions, resulting in a series of pollutants different from the original emissions, thus causing more serious secondary pollution.

(2) Air pollution is carcinogenic

Human beings can't live without air every second during their lifetime. Air pollution can cause many diseases, especially respiratory diseases, including the most severe lung cancer.

At the beginning of the 20th century, lung cancer mainly occurred in a few mines, mining and smelting occupational environment. After the First World War, lung cancer mortality began to rise. In the late 1930s, with the development of modern industry, atmospheric pollution, occupational carcinogens, tobacco and cigarette production or consumption soared, male patients in western industrialized countries experienced rapid lung cancer mortality. The mortality rate of lung cancer in the

UK was 10/10 million in 1930; 53/100,000 in 1950; 99.7/100,000 in 1966; and 120.3/100,000 in 1975. It has increased 12 times in the 45 years from 1930 to 1975.

In the United States from 1934 to 1974, male lung cancer jumped from the fifth leading cause to death, and its mortality increased from 3.0/100,000 to 54.5/10, a 17-fold increase; female lung cancer moved from the eighth to the top three, and died. The rate increased from 2/100,000 to 12.4/100,000, an increase of 5.2 times.

By the early 1980s, lung cancer in 24 countries and regions including the United Kingdom, France, the Netherlands, Germany, and North America was listed as the leading cause of death in patients with malignant tumors. Since the middle of the 20th century, the rapid rise of lung cancer in the western industrialized countries has been formed.

In industrialized countries, harmful gases such as power generation, steelmaking, automobiles, airplanes, fuel, energy, and large amounts of smoke are released into the atmosphere, polluting the air, and people are inhaled into the respiratory tract to cause an increase in the incidence and mortality of lung cancer.

2. Water pollution in environmental pollution and cancer

(1) Water pollution

a. Water is essential for the basic human life, because 63% of the body composition is water. The human body needs at least 1800ml of water per day. The cleanliness of water affects human health. The basic conditions for healthy drinking water are clear, refreshing, odorless, odor-free, and harmful substance.

b. The standards for drinking water determined by the state are:

Chromaticity <15 degrees, turbidity <3 degrees, pH between 6.5 and 8.5, iron <0.3 mg/L, Manganese <0.1 mg / L, zinc <1.0 mg / L, oxide <250 mg / L, phenols <0.002 mg / L.

Other indicators of toxic substances are lead <0.05mg/L and cadmium <0.01mg/L, Mercury <0.001 mg / L, arsenic <0.05 mg / L, selenium <0.01 mg / L.

The criteria for bacteria are:

The total number of cells was <100 cells/mg and E. coli <3 cells/L.

c. Source of water pollution:

Human beings are inseparable from water all the time in production activities and life. The pollution of water quality is mainly caused by industrial and agricultural production and urban sewage. In China, industrial pollution has intensified due to the rapid development of township and village enterprises. According to the survey, many key rivers are increasingly polluted. Fertilizers, pesticides and pesticides in agricultural production cause serious pollution of water quality.

The development of modern industry and the large-scale use of chemical fertilizers in agriculture have made environmental pollution increasingly serious and even affected the safety of drinking water. The famous Rhine in Europe has caused the disappearance of fish in the river due to industrial pollution. Seventy-five percent of the industrial water along the Volga River is discharged into the river without treatment, and most of the rivers in Asia are polluted, making it a highly degraded river in the world.

Some rural areas in China have the habit of using ditch pond water. A study in Qidong County, Jiangsu Province found that high incidence of liver cancer in this area is related to drinking pond water. Similar reports have been made in Fusui County, Guangxi. This indicates that water pollution is associated with high incidence of liver cancer. In Haining City, Zhejiang Province it was also found that the risk of colon cancer in drinking pond water was more than 7 times higher than that of drinking water.

d. What pollution is there in the water?

There are many types of pollution in the water, including microorganisms, heavy metals, and various chemical substances. Pesticides, fertilizers and pesticides are among the important pollutants in water, such as DDT, BHC and other chlorine-containing pesticides and polychlorinated biphenyls, etc., such chlorides are quite stable, and the damage is also lasting. In particular, the phosphate system in the detergent is often used in combination with the alkaline component, thus causing a red tide that is obviously polluted in the lake, the inland sea, and the river bay, causing fish to suffocate, and plankton and algae to be deformed. Water pollution not only has a fatal impact on aquatic life, but also enriches certain carcinogens. Therefore, it is possible to indirectly introduce the occurrence of cancer in the human body through the food chain.

In recent years, due to advances in water quality analysis technology, it has been found that more than 100 kinds of organic substances in water are carcinogenic, cancer-promoting and mutagenic. It has been confirmed in animal experiments that the following compounds can be added to drinking water to cause liver cancer: hexachlorocyclohexane, carbon tetrachloride, chloroform, trichloro and tetrachloroethylene, trichloroethane, and the like. In addition, some freshwater algae toxins, such as blue-green algae, have been found to have a significant effect on liver cancer.

The Sangde fish pond area in Shunde, Foshan, Guangdong Province is low-lying, easy to accumulate water, and the water pollution is serious. Residents have a high incidence of liver cancer, while neighboring Siping residents drink deep well water, have good water quality, and the incidence of liver cancer is relatively low. According to a large number of research data from the World Health Organization and the International Association for Research on Cancer, drinking substandard water can induce or promote cancer. Tests have shown that drinking water which contains more nickel is more susceptible to oral cancer, throat cancer and colorectal cancer; it is prone to esophageal cancer, laryngeal cancer and lung cancer with a large amount of cadmium or it is prone to stomach cancer, colon cancer, ovarian cancer and various lymphomas with more lead chemical element including ; more iron and zinc chemical element containing is prone to esophageal cancer.

3. Soil pollution in environmental pollution and cancer

In recent decades, a large amount of industrial waste water, waste slag and pesticides and fertilizers have been injected into the soil, which has deteriorated soil quality and accumulated poisons, especially around the factory, near cities and in sewage areas, and the soil is particularly polluted.

Soil contaminants are solid and liquid. Liquids often seep into the ground or flow with rain, etc., or evaporate and scatter with the wind.

However, solid contaminants remain in the soil for a long time.

The easily decomposed pollutants such as phenol and chlorine emitted from the factory are generally not easy to accumulate, and most of them are decomposed by microorganisms.

Organic substances from urban polluted water, although many types, can be naturally degraded. The most problematic soil pollutants are heavy metals such as mercury, arsenic, lead, cadmium, chromium, copper, etc. Once they enter the soil, they are difficult to decompose and difficult to remove. It may also accumulate year-round, with serious consequences. In addition to sewage and waste from factories and cities, soil pollutants can also come from dust in the atmosphere, which first pollutes the atmosphere and then settles to the ground to contaminate the soil. In China's energy consumption structure Coal consumption accounts for 3/4, causing pollution from coal burning, which the health and ecological impacts cannot be ignored. Waste from the nuclear industry and the atomic energy industry can increase radioactive materials in the soil, which are a threat to human health. It is also a carcinogenic factor.

4. Environmental chemical pollution and cancer

Chemical carcinogenesis

A chemical carcinogen refers to a chemical substance that induces tumor formation.

The problem of chemical carcinogenesis in the middle of the 20th century has caused widespread concern, mainly because of the increasing incidence of morbidity and mortality in modern times. The age of cancer is younger, and environmental chemical contamination is found to be closely related to the incidence of cancer. The World Health Organization has also pointed out that 80-90% of human cancers are related to environmental factors, mainly chemical factors.

The following are chemical substances that have been researched and proven to be carcinogenic

Vinyl chloride:

In 1974, people began to realize that this substance is the cause of occupational cancer.

In the experimental study of the experimental animals exposed to vinyl chloride it was found that liver cancer, brain cancer, kidney cancer, lung cancer and cancer of the lymphatic system existed in these animal. Or in the experimental studies, liver cancer, kidney cancer, lung cancer, and cancer of the lymphatic system were found in experimental animals exposed to vinyl chloride. However, the personnel concerned failed to recognize the hazards of these substances in a timely manner from these important experimental results, and thus failed to take timely measures to protect workers. Until recently, it just begun

The prohibition of the use of vinyl chloride sprays, plastic factories. It also changed the production process to prevent workers from being exposed. It needs to be pointed out in here that Vinyl chloride is an important raw material for records, packaging materials, medical test tubes, household appliances, bathroom equipment and many other plastic products. Plastic products are not inherently dangerous, but workers at vinyl chloride plants are 200 times more likely to get liver cancer than the average person.

Benzene:

This is a harmful chemical that destroys the hematopoietic function of the bone marrow. Aplastic anemia can occur in repeated exposure to benzene. This disease can become leukemia after a long time. In 1928, the first case of "benzene leukemia" was discovered.

Other countries have also shown that benzene is an occupational hazard, and Italian scientists reported 200 years ago that the risk of leukemia in printers and shoe factories is 20 times higher than in the general population.

Organic carcinogens, environmental pollution, polycyclic aromatic hydrocarbons carcinogens

Polycyclic aromatic hydrocarbons (PAFf) are a series of polycyclic aromatic hydrocarbon compounds produced by incomplete combustion of coal, petroleum, coal tar, and tobacco. Many of them have carcinogenic effects. It is a widely distributed class of environmental carcinogens and currently in the total number of 1000 multiple carcinogens polycyclic aromatic hydrocarbons account for more than 1/3.

In recent years, a large number of investigations have shown that air, water, soil, plants, etc. are contaminated by PAH.

The exhaust gas discharged from various motor vehicles such as automobiles and airplanes also contains a considerable amount of polycyclic aromatic hydrocarbons. Therefore, in the streets where traffic is frequent, the pollution of non-aromatic hydrocarbons on environmental carcinogens is also quite serious.

With the development of industry, the problem of carcinogenic polycyclic aromatic hydrocarbons has attracted more and more attention.

Certain activities and certain hobbies in human daily life are often closely related to environmental carcinogen polycyclic aromatic hydrocarbons. Smoking produces polycyclic aromatic hydrocarbons, which are important factors in inducing human lung cancer; in the fried, burning, and smoking of fats and oils, there are also carcinogenic polycyclic aromatic hydrocarbons. It is a carcinogen that poses a great threat to human health. We must pay enough attention to it.

In addition, benzopyrene in asphalt and hot asphalt is associated with a high incidence of cancer among road workers and roof workers. Agricultural workers are exposed to a variety of pesticides, herbicides and fertilizers, some are known human carcinogens, some have been induced cancer in experimental animals, and some have been proved to be mutagens after short-term tests. Pesticides enter the food chain and often accumulate in biological systems.

5. Physical factors in environmental pollution and cancer

(1) Ionizing radiation

With the development of science and technology, the frequent tests of nuclear tests, the application of nuclear energy and radioisotopes are increasing, and the amount of radioactive substances entering the human environment is also increasing. Therefore, the environmental pollution caused by ionizing radiation has received more and more attention.

What is called ionizing radiation?

Ionizing radiation refers to certain radioactive materials that emit radiation during the metamorphosis process, which can give the absorbing material a sufficient amount of energy to ionize the atoms and molecules. Some ionizing radiation is electromagnetic radiation, such as x-rays and r-rays.

Sources of ionizing radiation in human living environments:

a. Natural sources include cosmic rays and earth rays.

b. Artificial radiation sources have nuclear tests that increase environmental radioactive contamination. Nuclear fuel is mined, processed and reprocessed, such as ore mining, with radon and radioactive dust polluting the atmosphere. Due to energy shortages in nuclear power plants, more and more countries are developing nuclear power plants. This nuclear power industry has radioactive waste gas, waste water and waste slag, which will pollute the environment if not handled properly.

The use of isotopes, the application of isotopes in industry, agriculture and medicine, produces radioactive waste that can also pollute the environment.

The effects of ionizing radiation on the human body:

The body or Physical injury:

Such as chronic radiation sickness, malignant tumor, cataract, fertility decline.

(1) Radiation carcinogenesis, its carcinogenic effect has a long incubation period, such as leukemia, skin cancer, lung cancer, bone cancer.

(2) Genetic damage, causing hereditary diseases to occur in descendants.

Then how to prevent and control ionizing radiation pollution?

In order to protect the health of residents, the radioactive pollutants in the environment should not exceed the prescribed standards, the following measures must be taken:

(1) The site of the nuclear enterprise should be selected in a relatively dense population, the meteorological and hydrological conditions are conducive to the dilution and dilution of wastewater, exhaust gas, and areas with low seismic intensity to ensure the radiation exposure of residents in normal operation and accidents. The amount is low.

(2) The selection of process flow and equipment selection should consider the amount of waste generated and safe and reliable operation.

(3) Purification of wastewater and waste gas, and strict control of emissions and emission concentrations of radionuclides.

(4) Monitoring around nuclear companies and areas that may be exposed to radioactive contamination.

(5) For medical and scientific research workers and workers in related industries, the awareness of prevention of ionizing radiation should be strengthened, and radiation protection clothing and protective devices should be worn as much as possible.

(6) For ordinary residents, they should be as far away as possible from nuclear factories and nuclear power plants, do not drink the surrounding water sources, maintain a good mentality and scientific prevention.

6. Carcinogens that enter food from environmental pollution

With the development of science and technology, the food processing process is increasingly industrialized, and the external environment or the manufacturing process itself may cause various foreign substances, including chemical and biological carcinogens to contaminate food.

In the processing of food raw materials, artificial additives are added, and smoking, frying, baking, etc. are employed, and as a result, carcinogenic hybrids may occur in the food.

Food products are often stored and transported to reach consumers, thus providing an additional source of carcinogen-contaminated food.

Studying the sources of carcinogens on human food and how to eliminate such pollution is a very important issue.

(2) Relationship between lifestyle and cancer

Conduct research on cancer control and prevention and develop cancer control plans and measures

There are 1.6 million people suffering from cancer each year in China, and 1.3 million people die of cancer every year, and cancer patients are increasing at a rate of 3% each year. Preventing cancer, changing bad lifestyles, and developing a healthy lifestyle are imminent!

If you always maintain a healthy lifestyle, cancer may be difficult to invade because most of the cancers that are currently present are caused by unhealthy lifestyles and lifestyle behaviors. Therefore, the medical community reminds people to pay attention to their own lifestyle and to abandon bad habits.

Why connect lifestyle with cancer prevention?

Everyone has a proto-oncogene and the anti-cancer gene. Under normal circumstances, they are all in a state of sequestration. However, if a special situation occurs, the proto-oncogene is activated or the anti-cancer gene is lost, and people will develop cancer. How is the proto-oncogene activated and how is the anti-cancer gene lost? It must be related to external factors, which are derived from people's lifestyles and life behaviors. Therefore, lifestyle changes can indeed change the probability of cancer occurring.

1. Smoking, drinking and cancer

(1) Smoking and cancer

Smoking has become one of the serious social problems in the world today. There are 3 million people who die from smoking every year in the world, that is, on average, about 1 in 10 seconds, one person is killed by smoking.

There are at least 500,000 people who die of tobacco every year in our country. "A cigarette after a meal is better than a living god", "morning tea, night wine and smoking after meal". Smoking people always look for various excuses for swallowing cloud and throwing fog themselves. In fact, smoking has a lot of harm and no benefit. After burning and decomposing, cigarettes can release a variety of substances, of which hundreds of substances are harmful to the human body.

Smoking is closely related to cancer. Someone said: "When you order a cigarette, you put the cancer into your life." The incidence of cancer in smokers is 7 to 11 times higher than that of non-smokers, especially lung cancer is more closely related to smoking. About 80% of lung cancers are caused by long-term smoking. About 12% of smokers who smoke more than 25 cigarettes a day will develop lung cancer, and those who smoke 2 packs a day will definitely get lung cancer.

(1) Harmful ingredients of smoke

Toxic substances in tobacco include carcinogens and cancer-promoting substances. Among them, nicotine is a substance that is obviously toxic and carcinogenic.

1. Nicotine, also known as "nicotine."

Nicotine has an addictive effect similar to heroin and cocaine and is a major source of addiction. The amount of nicotine in the smoke is high and the toxicity is also high. The lethal dose is 40-60 mg, and a cigarette contains about 17 mg of nicotine. Nicotine quickly enters the lungs when smoking, and reaches the brain tissue with blood circulation for 7 seconds, reaching the body tissues for 20 seconds, making smokers achieve a pleasant feeling. Nicotine causes the central nervous system to begin to excite and then inhibit.

Nicotine also promotes the formation of cancer.

2. Filter, a cigarette filter made of polypropylene as a raw material, may have adverse effects on health. The United Nations International Agency for Cancer was discussed at a meeting to classify propylene as a "possible carcinogen."

3. Tobacco tar is a brown-yellow viscous resin commonly known as "oily smoke". It is produced when the cigarette is lit, and contains a variety of carcinogens and cancer-promoting substances such as polycyclic aromatic and its amines, phenols, ketones (formaldehyde, acetaldehyde).

4. Benzo[a]pyrene is a strong carcinogen. If the benzo[a]pyrene content in the air increases by 1 microgram/1000 cubic meter, the incidence of lung cancer will increase by 5% to 15%. In a burning pack of cigarettes, 2.4 to 2.8 micrograms of benzo[a]pyrene can be produced. It has a long-term and stimulating effect on bronchial epithelial cells and lung tissue cells, which will cause internal changes in these cells and lead to the direction of the development of cancer cells and eventually cause lung cancer.

5. Radioactive material.

For a person who smokes 20 cigarettes a day, the amount of radiation inhaled by a year is equivalent to 300 x-rays taken in 1 year.

6. Nitrosamine is a very strong carcinogen.

Tobacco produces a tobacco-specific nitrosamine during fermentation and when ignited. Scientists use this nitrosamine to treat hamsters and induce lung and bronchial cancer in mice.

(2) Cancer caused by smoking

A large number of animal experiments and epidemiological investigations have confirmed that smoking can lead to a variety of cancers, which are easily caused by lung cancer.

The incidence of oral and esophageal cancer in smokers is 4 to 5 times higher than that of non-smokers. People who are often squatting are also prone to develop lip cancer or people who often smoke pipes are also prone to lip cancer. Smokers' pancreatic cancer, bladder cancer, penile cancer, liver cancer, and leukemia all show an upward trend. Eating and drinking while smoking makes toxic substances swallow into the stomach and cause stomach cancer.

(3) The harm of female smoking

Smoking is more harmful to women. It will destroy the active function of the body's immune system to some extent, so it may increase the risk of uterine cancer in women who smoke through the interaction of human papillomavirus or other viruses.

(4) Cancer risk of passive smoking

It is worth noting that many non-smokers have become passive smokers because they live among smokers. If the husband smokes and his wife does not smoke, his wife is more likely to develop lung cancer than her husband does not smoke. Smoking not only harms self, but also harms the closest people. Whether the smoker is willing to believe or not willing to admit it, all of it is true.

It has been confirmed that smoking is related to cancer. Smoking has become a public hazard, and the World Health Organization has decided to write May 31 of each year as a "smoke-free day" to promote global action and work together to reduce the health risks of tobacco.

There are regulations in China that prohibit smoking in various public places. Smoking is an expression of no knowledge.

(5) Drinking and cancer

Human drinking has a history of thousands of years. From a medical point of view, the main ingredient in wine is ethanol (commonly known as "alcohol"). But if you indulge in the spirits all day long, it is very harmful to the body. It turns out that alcoholics are prone to cancer.

Therefore, whether wine is good or harmful to people or not, is depending on the size of the amount. A small amount of alcohol is good for the human body. Drinking a lot of alcohol can cause symptoms such as alcoholism and confusion. And will damage the various systems of the body, causing a variety of cancers

1). harmful substances in the wine

The chemical composition of the wine is extremely complicated, but the content of acetaldehyde is high. The aldehyde is a kind of harmful substance in the wine. The ugliness of people in drunkenness is mainly caused by acetaldehyde. Mild alcoholism is manifested by the excitement of the central nervous system, and in severe cases, it is suppressed. Long-term excessive drinking can cause chronic alcoholism, mainly manifested by decreased response, dementia, and dullness.

2). The causes of alcohol-induced cancer

For decades, people have clinically recognized that alcoholism has a certain relationship with the emergence of certain cancers. Strictly speaking, drinking is not the direct cause of illness, but drinking is an inducer or promoter of carcinogens and can inhibit the function of the immune system. Alcohol itself is not a carcinogenic substance. Animal experiments have shown that only alcohol and certain chemical carcinogens or procarcinogens are given to animals at the same time. Alcohol can cause carcinogenic effects on certain organs under certain conditions. But we still can't take it lightly.

Alcohol has an inhibitory effect on immune function, and inhibition of immunity is often an important cause of tumorigenesis. Alcohol does not directly cause cancer, but long-term alcohol abuse can be a cofactor for the development of liver cancer through a variety of indirect pathways.

3). drinking can induce cancer

In recent years, a large number of epidemiological studies have confirmed that alcohol abuse is associated with the occurrence of multiple cancers. According to a survey conducted by an American authority, alcohol is associated with the development of breast cancer, colon cancer, thyroid tumor, and malignant melanoma. It has been reported that women drinking alcohol can increase breast cancer by 20% to 60%, thyroid tumors by 20% to 70%, and skin cancer by 20% to 70%.

The risk of oral and throat tumors in drinking high-concentration drinkers is 12 times higher than that of the average person.

4). drinking advice

In summary, excessive drinking is harmful to the human body.

Therefore, give advice to those who are indulging in spirits throughout the day:

Drinking must be controlled, especially those with hepatitis and cirrhosis should resolutely stop drinking. Alcoholics can drink 2 cups a day (about 50 ml of wine, 25 degrees of alcohol, such as wine) or less, and must quit smoking when drinking. Women do not drink alcohol during pregnancy.

Synergistic effect of tobacco and alcohol

Some people in foreign countries have used a case-control study to examine the effects of smoking and drinking, both smoking and drinking on cancer.

The results showed or it was turned out:

The toxicity of both tobacco and wine has a synergistic effect, and the risk of cancer among tobacco and alcohol users will multiply. Both smoking and drinking, the incidence of cancer is more than 15 times higher than the general population.

The international community has formed a more consistent view:

Alcohol and tobacco have synergistic effects that increase the risk of cancer.

2, household goods, office supplies and cancer

(1) Household appliances

1). electromagnetic radiation

With the increasing modernization of society, a large number of household appliances have flooded into the family. Household appliances generate electromagnetic waves of various wavelengths and frequencies, forming electromagnetic pollution that threatens people's health. Scientists recently published a report that many home appliances generate electromagnetic radiation that exceeds safety standards. Excessive use of home appliances may cause cancer, Parkinson's disease, Alzheimer's disease and other diseases. An authoritative organization in the United States has reported and recommended that the safety standard for magnetic induction generated by electromagnetic radiation should not exceed a certain value, otherwise it may cause diseases such as cancer. According to the report, the magnetic field induction intensity near the commonly used vacuum cleaner is 100 times the safety standard, the electric drill is 50 times, and the blower is 35 times. Therefore, we should not use these appliances for a long time. For another example, scientists have conducted microwave radiation tests on mice and found that their white blood cells proliferate irregularly, which is very similar to the white blood cell proliferation produced by blood cancer. In other words, microwaves can cause cancer. Therefore, when using a microwave oven, the operator should try to leave the furnace body at least 1 meter away from the furnace to protect it from electromagnetic waves.

2). TV

Watching TV has become an indispensable part of people's daily lives. However, watching TV should also pay attention to science and pay attention to physical health. Otherwise, it will be harmful to the body and mind.

3). fluorescent screen

Recently, a foreign survey also pointed out that many devices with fluorescent screens, such as computers and televisions, produce a toxic gas called brominated dibenzofuran. Prolonged, close contact may cause cancer. In order to prevent the generation of these toxic gases, such electrical appliances should be repaired in time if they are faulty, and they should not be allowed to "work with disease". When using them, they can maintain indoor air circulation.

(2) Office appliances

1) Copier

Modern offices are often inseparable from photocopiers, but they can produce potential carcinogens.

Several possible sources are:

1). The oxygen in the air generates ozone under the action of the high voltage of the copying machine. Ozone is a gas that has a fishy smell and may be an inducer and a carcinogen. When smelling the smell of ozone, you should find a way to ventilate the office environment.

2). Copying toner in the copier is also a potential carcinogen. This powder is made of carbon powder, which contains contaminants, but is also a mutagen and a possible carcinogen.

3). "Carbon-free" copy papers contain PCBs or formaldehyde, which is an irritating potential carcinogen. Avoid using such papers.

2) Home decoration

With the improvement of living conditions, many families have to make some renovations after they have housing. Because the novel decoration materials include carcinogens such as aromatics and formaldehyde, some decorative materials also have certain radioactive substances (such as sputum), which have certain promotion effects on cancer production. Especially children, their ability to withstand environmental pollution is weak. According to reports, the incidence of childhood leukemia has increased year by year in recent years.

Some experts believe that the increase in the incidence rate is closely related to family decoration, especially luxury decoration. Because the toxic substances and radioactive materials in the decoration materials have not been exhausted, it is definitely harmful to the body to move in and live immediately, especially for children with delicate constitution.

(3) Inferior cleaning supplies

Benzene is a commonly used chemical solvent commonly used in household cleaners, stain removers, and solvents. Gasoline also contains benzene. It contains benzene from adhesives for shoemaking to pesticides, inks and paints. Benzene poses a risk of leukemia. Prolonged exposure to benzene is more dangerous and should avoid the use of detergents containing carcinogens such as carbon tetrachloride and perchloroethylene.

(4) Other carcinogens in the family

Carcinogens, usually from household items, such as pesticides, cosmetics, household plastics and rubber products, and carcinogens from foods such as bacon, pickles, fried foods, etc., have gradually caused widespread pay attention to it. However, there are some little-known carcinogens that have not caught people's attention. These unattractive family carcinogens mainly include:

1). Carcinogens from tap water:

American researchers found that a bactericide-bleach powder added to tap water will release active chlorine. Drinking tap water with active chlorine for a long time may induce bladder cancer and rectal cancer.

2). paper can cause cancer:

Foreign scientists have discovered that the paper that people use every day is also one of the carcinogens. Some people use used newspapers and magazines to wrap food. These waste newspapers have black ink printed words. The ink materials used in the printing plant basically contain toxic substances such as benzene, toluene, xylene, polyvinyl chloride, paste resin and the like. Packing food with used newspapers can easily contaminate food and cause harm to the human body. According to reports, some toxins can cause cancer of human cells.

3. Cosmetics and Cancer

Cosmetics enrich people's lives, but they may also bring certain harm to human health. From the perspective of long-term effects, their carcinogenic toxicity must be vigilant.

(1) Carcinogenic materials in cosmetics

In cosmetic raw materials, the problem with additives is particularly prominent. Arsenic, a common toxic substance in cosmetic raw materials, has the effect of causing skin cancer. Most of the fragrances and pigments contained in cosmetics are synthetic products made from coal tar, and some of them have carcinogenic effects. For example, the alkaline ruthenium in the lipstick, the blush in the blush, and the flame red have strong carcinogenicity; creamy yellow has been shown to cause liver cancer; pigment amaranth has also been reported to cause bowel cancer. For example, nitrite as a preservative is widely used in various cosmetics, and is a precursor of a strong carcinogen nitrosamine.

(2) Cosmetic production process and cancer

Various carcinogens may be introduced into the raw materials of cosmetics, and new carcinogens may be mixed in the production process of cosmetics.

(3) Carcinogenic pathways of cosmetics

The way cosmetics enter the body is mainly absorbed by the skin, and can also be absorbed through the digestive tract or the respiratory tract. Lipstick can be absorbed through the skin, or through the lips, water, and eating. Eyelid cream and cream contain talcum powder, often mixed with carcinogen asbestos. When used, it will overflow into the air and cause lung cancer with breathing into the lungs.

Some data indicate that hair dyes can cause carcinogenic effects on the human body.

Under normal circumstances, if you use hair dye for 10 years, the human skin only absorbs l%, this substance can cause cancer, such as bladder cancer, kidney cancer and skin cancer.

The National Cancer Institute uses animal hair dyes such as aminotoluene, which is used as an animal experiment. Now, the mice tested have tumors in their skin, liver, thyroid, lymph nodes and genital system. After long-term research, many experts in the US anti-cancer organization have confirmed that male hair dyes have a greater risk of suffering from blood cancer, and the longer the hair dyeing time, the greater the risk of suffering from blood cancer. The incidence of blood cancer in hairdressers is also higher than that of the average person. A large number of studies have confirmed that dyes are carcinogenic.

4. Clothing and Cancer

(1) Clothing

Since the garment manufacturer performs anti-wrinkle and shrink-proof treatment on the cotton fiber fabric, it is to add a formaldehyde resin coating. It is combined with the molecular chain of cotton fiber under high temperature and high pressure, and there is a sense of stiffness. If the cleaning is not clean in the later stage, the formaldehyde monomer can be released from the cloth and adsorbed on the surface of the cloth. If people buy this fashion new clothes for a long time to wear it without washing it first, one is to directly stimulate the skin to cause cancer, and the other is to release formaldehyde with a pungent odor and cause cancer.

(2) bra

Bras have become an indispensable part of modern women's underwear. However, if the bra is worn improperly, it will lead to the formation of breast cancer, so it must be used with caution. According to the findings of the American Institute of Diseases, women who wear bras for a long time are prone to breast cancer, especially women who wear bras for more than 12 hours a day, have a breast cancer rate of 75 ‰ and bras no more than 12 hours. Women have a probability of 0.5%.

The study also found that Japanese women have a lower probability of developing breast cancer because they do not have the habit of wearing a bra. The proportion who suffer this disease of American women who like to wear bras is high in the world. The reason why wearing a bra is easy to cause cancer is that the bra compresses the chest, hinders the normal circulation of the lymph in the breast, and wears the bra for a long time to block the harmful metabolic production of the cells. Over time, the normal cells there will become pathological. To this end, experts warned women that it should not wear a bra as much as possible. When buying a bra, it would rather buy the bigger and not the smaller. It is better not to wear bras more than 12 hours. The bras should not be worn for more than 12 hours a day, or wearing bras is no more than 12 hours a day.

The facts that have been observed so far,

It shows that living habits are factors that can not be ignored in the study of the cause of cancer. To this end, experts warned women that they should wear bras as much as possible;

When buying a bra, don't be too small; wear a bra every day for no more than 12 hours.

The facts that have been observed so far indicate that lifestyle habits are factors that cannot be ignored in the study of the etiology of cancer. However, due to the complexity of living habits, it is difficult to make a clear conclusion about its causal relationship with tumors. Therefore, the above-mentioned various facts can only be regarded as an apocalyptic data. The exact relationship and the mechanism of inducing tumors require in-depth research in the future. Strengthen publicity and education on the relationship between "life habits" and cancer, so that the masses can understand relevant knowledge and gradually correct some unhealthy living habits and stay away from cancer.

(3) Relationship between diet and cancer

Patients in the oncology clinic often ask the physician a question: which foods can't be eaten? which foods can be eaten? what is the "forbidden mouth"?

This is a question worthy of attention.

There are two important measures to prevent cancer. One is to avoid contact with carcinogenic factors, and the other is to eat foods that can prevent cancer. Therefore, it is a problem worthy of attention. Diet is one of the most important factors in lifestyle, and it is important to prevent cancer by improving lifestyle.

The occurrence of cancer requires a long process. Sometimes it takes years. In this long time, the two forces are fighting each other. On the one hand, it is carcinogenic and cancer-promoting factors. On the other hand, it is a cancer suppressor.

The former has a greater effect than the latter, and the human body is prone to cancer. The latter's role is greater than the former, the human body is not easy to get cancer. Most of the carcinogenic, cancer-promoting and cancer prevention factors come from diet. Therefore, people in the diet enhance the role of cancer suppression, reduce carcinogenic and cancer-promoting factors, thereby achieving the purpose of diet prevention.

Natural foods containing cancer promoters or carcinogens include tannins, ferns, baicalein, cycads, sorghum, persimmon, coconut, and betel nut have higher tannin content, chewing betel nuts containing tannins is prone to oral cancer and a wolf in fern can cause bowel cancer, bladder cancer and lung cancer in animal experiments.

Natural foods also contain a number of cancer suppressing factors, such as cruciferous vegetables, citrus, soybeans, tomatoes, garlic, radishes, mushrooms, asparagus, bitter gourd, eggplant, garlic and so on.

Diet refers to drinks and food:

First, the drink

(a) water

1. Water pollution

Water is essential for basic human life because 63% of the body composition is water, and the body needs to supplement at least 1800ml of water per day.

The cleanliness of water affects human health.

The drinking water standards set by the state are:

Chromaticity <15 degrees; Turbidity <3 degrees; PH is between 6.5 and 8.5; Iron <0.3mg/L, Manganese <0.1mg/L, Zinc <1.0mg,

Oxide <250ml/L, Phenols <0.002mg/L, Other indicators of toxic substances are lead <0.05mg/L, Cadmium <0.01mg/L, Mercury <0.001mg/L, Arsenic <0.05mg/L, Selenium <0.01mg/L; the total number of bacteria <100 / mg, E. coli <3 / L.

The development of modern industry and the large-scale use of chemical fertilizers in agriculture have made environmental pollution increasingly serious and even affected the safety of drinking water. The famous Rhine in Europe has caused the disappearance of fish in the river due to industrial pollution. 75% of the industrial wastewater along the Volga River is discharged into the river without treatment. Most of the rivers in Asia are polluted and become the most degraded rivers in the world.

A study in Qidong County, Jiangsu Province, found that the high incidence of liver cancer in this area is related to drinking ditch soil. A similar report has been published in Fusui County, Guangxi, indicating that water pollution is associated with high incidence of liver cancer. In Haining City, Zhejiang Province it was also found that the risk of colon cancer in drinking pond water was more than 7 times higher than that of drinking water.

2. The relationship between water pollution and cancer

In recent years, due to advances in water quality analysis, it has been found that there are more than 100 kinds of organic substances in water as carcinogenic, cancer-promoting and mutagenic. It has been confirmed in animal experiments that the following compounds can be added to drinking water to cause liver cancer: Hexachlorocyclohexane, carbon tetrachloride, chloroform, trichloro and tetrachloroethylene, trichloroethane, etc. In addition, some freshwater algae toxins, such as blue-green algae, have been found to have a significant effect on promoting liver cancer.

According to a large number of research data from the World Health Organization and the International Association for Research on Cancer, drinking substandard water can induce or promote cancer. Tests have shown that drinking water containing more nickel is prone to oral cancer and throat cancer. It is prone to esophageal cancer, laryngeal cancer, rectal cancer and lung cancer with a large amount of cadmium; more lead-containing chemical elements are prone to stomach cancer, intestinal cancer, ovarian cancer and various lymphomas; more iron and zinc chemical elements including are prone to esophageal cancer.

3, diet and cancer

In 217 AD, there was a philosopher in the Western Jin Dynasty called Fu Xuan. He wrote a book called "Mouth or Mingming", which put forward a famous saying: "The disease is from the mouth." Of course, he was referring to the reasons for the illness caused by improper diet, such as overeating, eating unclear food or contaminated water. Acute gastroenteritis is caused by taking unclean food or contaminated water.

Today, in the second decade of the 21st century, in the above-mentioned meaning of "sickness from the mouth", we also have to add the occurrence or incidence of some cancers, which are also related to improper diets. It may also mention the meaning of "cancer from mouth". "But it doesn't mean that all cancers are caused by diet. Such as, acute gastroenteritis is caused by overeating and overdrinking, taking unclean food or contaminated water.

According to experts, 30% to 35% of human cancers are due to improper diet. Of course, it is not that diet will definitely cause cancer. It should be said that a reasonable diet can help prevent cancer, which is called cancer prevention food.

However, both epidemiologists and clinicians have observed and confirmed that diets are indeed associated with specific cancers in different parts of the body.

However, whether an epidemiologist or a clinician has been observed and confirmed that the diet is indeed associated with specific cancers in different parts of the body.

(1) Digestive tract cancer

Since the diet is digested and absorbed through the digestive tract, both the food itself and its catabolic products are in close contact with the gastrointestinal tract. It can be said that they bear the brunt. The digestive tract includes the esophagus, stomach, small intestine, colon and rectum, as well as liver, gallbladder, pancreas, etc. The following is only the relationship between the pathogenesis and diet.

1). diet and esophageal cancer

From the current research of scientists, there are many factors that affect the occurrence of esophageal cancer:

a, Lack of vitamin A and vitamin C

In Linzhou City, Henan Province, a high incidence area for esophageal cancer in China, scientists have conducted nutrition surveys in different villages. It was found that Vitamin A is seriously deficient, and vitamin C in most areas is only 30% to 50% of the normal standard value.

b, lack of certain trace elements

Chinese scientists have also found that drinking water, food and vegetables in high-incidence areas of esophageal cancer are low in molybdenum, manganese, zinc and magnesium. The molybdenum, zinc, magnesium and other elements in the serum of local residents are also low.

c, pickled and mildewed food:

The nitrosamine chemical is a strong carcinogen that can cause a variety of tumors. Among them, dimethylamine and diethylnitrosamine and methylbenzylnitrosamine are found in marinated meat and fish, especially in crude fish sauce. In addition, among those of older and dry Radish, older cornmeal, sauerkraut and some mildewed food, even sausages and beer are more or less present. These are the diets that people in high-risk areas of esophageal cancer often eat.

Animal experiments have shown that they can induce tumors in animals such as rats, mice, rabbits, and even monkeys.

d, other factors related to diet:

The food is too hot and the food is too rough.

2). According to epidemiological studies, it may be related to the following factors:

a, delicious smoked food:

Due to the large amount of polycyclic hydrocarbons produced during the smoking process, including phenylpropanoids, which is a strong carcinogen that penetrates the entire food product during the smoking process and therefore contains a higher concentration. In addition, in some smoking operations, the temperature is very high, and the protein is easily decomposed to produce a mutagen at such a high temperature, especially during scorching, and also has a carcinogenic component.

b, nitrate in drinking water and food:

Scientists have conducted investigations many times and in several high-risk areas of gastric cancer. Nitrate and nitrite levels were found to be significantly higher in drinking water and in certain cereals in these areas than in low-incidence areas.

Nitrate and nitrite can form nitrite in the human stomach, which is a carcinogenic compound.

c, like to eat pickled food:

The high incidence of gastric cancer may be related to the frequent intake of salted fish and bacon. Salted fish and bacon contain more muscle fibers. It is possible that nitrosation in gastric juice forms carcinogenic nitrosomethylurea leading to gastric cancer. Studies have shown that high levels of trace elements such as lead, zinc, cobalt and chromium in food can also be associated with the pathogenesis of gastric cancer.

d, mildew food:

Chinese scientists surveyed high-risk areas of gastric cancer and found that food and eating material in these areas were seriously contaminated by molds and their toxins. Even in the gastric juice of patients with gastric cancer, molds and its toxins were detected.

e, drinking:

Alcoholism can burn the stomach mucosa, causing chronic gastritis, and gastritis may turn into gastric cancer.

f, gastric cancer is also associated with gastric ulcer, gastric polyps and Helicobacter pylori infection in the stomach.

g, eat more fruits and vegetables, rich in vitamin C, and milk play certain role in preventing gastric cancer.

3). Diet has a very close relationship with the occurrence of colon and rectal cancer and hereditary and precancerous lesions, but the diet also plays an extremely important role.

a, high fat diet:

Many surveys have shown that in high-fat diets, especially those who eat more sheep and beef fat, the incidence of colorectal cancer is significantly higher than that of people who eat low-fat diets, which has also been confirmed in animal experiments. It can be related to the production of more bile acids and cholesterol by fat metabolism. At the same time, a high-fat diet can also promote the growth of anaerobic bacteria in the intestinal lumen. Under the action, it will produce more carcinogenic ingredients.

b, insufficient dietary fiber:

In Africa, Finland, Japan, and China, people have more dietary fiber in their diet. Therefore, the incidence of colorectal cancer is significantly lower than that of European and American countries, which can be related to the rapid defecation and the high amount of feces, resulting in a short contact time between carcinogens and intestinal mucosa.

c, other dietary factors:

Eating more foods rich in vitamin A can reduce the incidence of colorectal cancer; people who drink more beer, or drink beer or other alcohol, have a higher incidence of colorectal cancer.

4). diet and liver cancer

Primary liver cancer (liver cancer), about 250,000 people die of liver cancer every year in the world, 40% of which are in China.

According to the study of diet and etiology, the incidence of liver cancer is related to diet. At present, many studies have been done on the etiology of liver cancer. In recent years, it has mainly focused on hepatitis B virus and dietary factors, and among dietary factors the attention has been paid to the contamination of mycotoxins and drinking water.

5). animal experiment results show that aflatoxin-containing feed can induce a variety of experimental cancers, mainly liver cancer. The extent or degree to which food is contaminated with aflatoxin is positively correlated with the incidence of liver cancer. In China's high incidence of liver cancer, in addition to mycotoxins, viral hepatitis and drinking water or lack of nutrition are factors that cannot be ignored.

In particular, 75% to 85% of patients with high incidence of liver cancer in China are accompanied by cirrhosis. And, mostly, it is complicated by massive nodular cirrhosis after hepatitis. Therefore, it has been suggested that hepatitis B virus infection and aflatoxin combined to cause liver cancer. Aflatoxin can inhibit cellular immunity and easily convert liver cirrhosis caused by hepatitis B virus into liver cancer.

In China, the main high-incidence areas of liver cancer have common characteristics, namely, drinking water pollution of residents, and the degree of drinking water pollution is positively correlated with the incidence of liver cancer. It is suggested that there may be carcinogens in the water source.

Long-term alcohol abuse can significantly damage liver cells and cause malnutrition. Liver cirrhosis is prone to occur in the liver, and liver cancer can be developed on the basis of cirrhosis.

(2) Breast cancer

The occurrence of breast cancer has a great relationship with endocrine. However, due to differences in diet, the incidence of breast cancer is very different, indicating that diet plays an important role in the occurrence of breast cancer.

A lot of data prove that there is a positive correlation between high-fat diet and breast cancer, especially with the increase in consumption of beef, mutton, pork and sweets. Perhaps this is one of the main reasons why the incidence of breast cancer in Westerners is much higher than in China.

Contrary to the above-mentioned high fat and high calorie, people who eat more vegetables and low-fat, low-protein diets have a lower incidence of breast cancer, and this woman has lower levels of estrogen in the blood. This may have a more direct relationship with breast cancer.

4, nutrients and cancer

Nutrition is the whole process of ingesting, digesting and absorbing food for the body to maintain life activities. Nutrition usually refers to six major nutrients, namely carbohydrates, protein, fat, vitamins, minerals and trace elements, water. These elements are the material basis in the life process, and the normal metabolic activities that sustain life are indispensable. In general, nutrients in natural conditions in natural foods do not cause cancer by themselves. However, in the human body, if the nutrients are dysfunctional, too much or too little may have a cancer-promoting effect. Epidemiological investigations have shown that a variety of nutrients, especially fat, promote cancer. Of course, there are also many nutrients that have an inhibitory effect on cancer.

Fat and cancer

The current consensus is that a high-fat diet can promote colon and breast cancer.

The intake of animal fat is directly proportional to the incidence and mortality of these two types of cancer. According to a survey of dozens of countries, the higher the amount of meat, the higher the mortality rate of breast, colon and prostate cancer. Studies have also shown that the higher the fat intake per person per day, the higher the mortality rate of breast and colon cancer. Chinese people are used to rice, corn, and beans.

The incidence of colon cancer and breast cancer is lower than that of Europeans and Americans. In the epidemiological survey of the population, it was found that the risk of breast cancer increased significantly when the daily intake of fat was above 80 grams. Case-control surveys of colon cancer have similar results. Experts agree that colon cancer and breast cancer can be prevented by controlling diet structure, especially reducing fat content in food.

In addition, leukemia, leukopenia, rectal cancer and ovarian cancer are also significantly associated with dietary fat intake, with the exception of gastric cancer; others believe that fat intake in the diet has a significant relationship with pancreatic cancer, and animal experiments support this argument. A large amount of unsaturated fat diet makes animals more susceptible to pancreatic cancer.

5, vitamins and cancer

Vitamins are a general term for a large class of organic nutrients necessary to maintain normal life activities.

Different types of vitamins have different structures and functions. Generally speaking, as long as a small amount can meet the daily physiological needs, insufficient or lack of intake can cause changes in the body's physiological functions, and even produce nutritional deficiencies. With the deepening of research on cancer prevention and control, people are increasingly aware that certain vitamins are closely related to the occurrence and development of many cancers.

Vitamin A, commonly known as retinoic acid, plays an important role in maintaining normal vision, epithelial integrity, growth and development. Many case-control studies have shown that certain epithelial cell carcinomas such as breast, lung, skin and stomach, as well as bowel and bladder cancer are associated with too little vitamin A intake. Vitamin A is mainly associated with lung cancer. Vitamin A and carotene come from green and yellow vegetables, certain fruits, whole milk and liver.

The latter can be converted to vitamin A after absorption to exert physiological functions. Therefore, those who eat the above foods often, the incidence of cancer is also low.

Vitamin C, commonly known as ascorbic acid, is named for its ability to prevent ascorbate. In the huge vitamin family, the cancer prevention effect of vitamin C can be considered as a leader, especially in the prevention of esophageal cancer and gastric cancer. Vitamin C can prevent the occurrence of experimental cancer through a variety of mechanisms, among which antioxidants are important. Population epidemiological surveys have shown that people with high intake of fresh vegetables and fruits have low incidence of cancer and low mortality, especially it is obvious in gastric cancer, the same is true for lung cancer, esophageal cancer, colon cancer, rectal cancer, breast cancer, and bladder cancer. The level of vitamin C in patients with cancer is significantly lower than in healthy people.

Vitamin E, also known as tocopherol, was named for its early discovery that it promotes the reproductive capacity of animals. The main role of the human body is to resist oxidation. Experts have found through animal experiments that vitamin E can prevent skin cancer in mice through its antioxidant effects.

In addition, vitamin E can inhibit the formation of nitrosamines in the stomach, so it can prevent the occurrence of gastric cancer. Vitamin E or C can be gotten through the food. Both have the function of blocking the formation of nitrosamines, which can reduce the incidence of gastric cancer. Vitamin E is mainly found in vegetable oils, grains and nuts, and there are few shortages or deficiency in our population.

Everything has its two sides, on the one hand, vitamins as a nutrient are essential for humans. On the other hand, the growth of cancer also requires a lot of vitamins. Therefore, in the process of cancer occurrence and development, the cancer-promoting effects of certain vitamins are often difficult to avoid. But what we can do is when using a metabolic antagonist, it try to avoid the use of this vitamin in large doses, or limit the intake of foods containing this vitamin, in order to improve the therapeutic effect of anticancer agents.

6. Food preservation and cooking and cancer

People must eat many kinds of food at the same time every day. According to modern nutrition research, carcinogenic substances may be present in food. Some foods contain natural carcinogens, and more are caused by environmental pollution.

(1) Improper preservation produces carcinogens

During pickling or salting animal food, in order to kill the bacteria or be bacteriostatic and keep color, it is often added nitrate or nitrite. Fish and livestock are rich in amines. The nitroso compound is easily synthesized under suitable conditions. The suitable conditions are acidic state, certain amine concentration, and microorganisms. Nitrosamines are found in fermented wine, fish sauce and pickles or pickles. Under anaerobic conditions, after the mold is contaminated, the original nitrate can form nitrosamines. **The toxicity of nitrosamines to humans is mainly liver damage, and it is also carcinogenic, teratogenic and mutagenic. When salting, it is necessary to add a large amount of salt, and the main component of salt is sodium chloride, but also contains a small amount of sodium nitrate and sodium nitrite. The nitrates entering the body are reduced to nitrite by** bacteria in the mouth and stomach. Then In the stomach it can have metabolism with protein to produce **an amine group to carry out nitrosation reaction, synthesis of nitrosamines with strong carcinogenic activity. It also converts methionine to ethionine to make some sterol chains become unsaturated. And produce polycyclic aromatic hydrocarbons, etc. These substances are all strong carcinogens. Among them, esophageal cancer and gastric cancer are more common.**

(2) Cooking and processing produces carcinogens

Foods can be lost, denatured, and even produce toxic and harmful substances due to improper processing methods.

For example, when fat is cooked, high temperature treatment such as fried and frying will form a toxic and harmful polymer. The latter is absorbed by the human body and then combined with the enzyme to deactivate the enzyme, which may cause the animal to grow stagnant and the liver to enlarge, reproductive function dysfunction and liver dysfunction, and even carcinogenic effects. Therefore, the grease should not be heated more than 150 ° C, and do not use it repeatedly, and use less fried and frying cooking methods.

The latter is absorbed by the body and bound to the enzyme, which makes the enzyme inactive, which may cause animal growth to stagnate, liver enlargement, reproductive function and liver dysfunction, and even carcinogenic effects.

Therefore, grease heating should generally not exceed 150 ° C, and do not use it repeatedly, and try to use fried, fried cooking methods. If the protein is heated too high and the time is too long, the amino acid will be oxidized, difficult to digest, and cannot be used. When the temperature is above 190 ° C, it is also possible to produce a mutagenic heterocyclic amine compound, which has a very strong carcinogenic effect. Fried salted fish and bacon can produce N-nitroso compounds.

1). smoked

Some people especially like roast duck, roast chicken, smoked fish, ham, sausage and other smoked food. In some areas, residents also eat foods that are grilled directly on the fire, such as roast lamb and roasted sweet potatoes. But we should not ignore the fact that: smoked foods contain carcinogens and are often consumed in large quantities to induce stomach and bowel cancer. Although smoking is a long-established food processing method in China, it also brings us many carcinogens.

In order to make the human body healthy, the old food that advises smoked food is to be restrained.

2). fried

The cooking process of fried foods is another source of carcinogens in addition to smoking. Various fats and oils are used for frying, and carcinogens can be produced when the temperature is too high.

The amino acids in the protein from fried foods and charred fish, meat, etc., can be decomposed under high temperature conditions to produce heterocyclic amines, such as tryptophan, which is more mutagenic than aflatoxin. At present, many experiments have shown that feeding animals with subcutaneous heat or subcutaneous injection can cause benign and malignant tumors. Overheated oils have a great toxic effect on animals and cause precancerous lesions of the gastric mucosa - polyps, ulcers, and chronic atrophic gastritis.

7, food additives and cancer

Food additive refers to a chemically synthesized or natural substance that is added and used during the production, processing, and storage of food. Its main purpose is to improve the sensory properties (color, aroma, taste, etc.) of foods. For example, adding pigments, spices, saccharin, etc. during the production of cold foods and drinks. To prevent the change of the color of the food during storage or transportation, it is to add a coloring agent, etc. Preservatives are added to control the growth of microorganisms and inhibit the growth of bacteria, so that foods have greater stability during storage; it is adding emulsifier, thickener, loosening agent, etc. according to the requirements of the food processing process; in order to improve the quality of food, the quality improvers an nutritional supplements, etc. are added. Although most of the above food additives are safe for the human body, some food additives do have carcinogenic activity. For example, improper use of a wide variety of food additives may cause some of the carcinogens to cause harm to the human body.

Nitrate and nitrous acid are long-lasting and effective color formers. Nitrite can not only be firmly bound to the 2 valent iron ion of myoglobin and makes it not be oxidized to 3 valent iron ion, and it will become stable and red nitrite and protein decomposition products. The amines (secondary amines) combine to form nitrosamines with strong carcinogenic effects.

Nitrosamine is currently recognized as a carcinogen in the world. According to animal experiments, not only long-term small-dose attacks have carcinogenic effects, but also a sufficient amount of impact, but also carcinogenic effects.

8, the preservatives

Preservatives are a type of additive, and many of the additives are synthetic chemicals, and some do cause cancer. It is generally prudent to use chemicals as additives in the world today. There are two types of preservatives that can be used in China: one type is benzoic acid and sodium benzoate; the other type is sorbic acid and potassium sorbate, which the application range areas are limited to soy sauce, vinegar, jam, sherbet, fruity dew, wine, sparkling wine, soda, low-salt pickles, candied fruit, hawthorn cake, canned food, etc.

Sorbic acid is a kind of preservative used in the world. It is an unsaturated fatty acid, which has strong inhibition and killing effect on fungi, and also inhibits bacteria and yeast. For example, in order to manufacture canned foods, sorbic acid is commonly used for preservation. At the 1956 Rome International Conference, it was included in the class of compounds that met safety standards. However, it has recently been reported that long-term subcutaneous injection of sorbic acid in rats causes the formation of fibrosarcoma. Therefore, it is better to eat less sorbic acid as a preservative before it is determined.

In addition, nitrate is added to fish and meat processing, mainly as a coloring agent, but also as a preservative such as bacon, sausage and ham. The amount of these salts added is strictly limited because such preservatives tend to become nitrosamines which have a strong causing- cancer effect for the intestinal and gastric cancers.

To ensure the health of the people, the country or the state regulates the amount of preservatives in various foods.

Despite this, attention must be paid to the amount of preservatives in the foods consumed.

9. Diet to prevent cancer

I often listens to my friends and say: "What strange diseases are there now, it's terrible, and many of them are eaten." This may sound a bit confusing. In fact, there are some truths or it does have some truth. Now with the continuous improvement of living standards, what you want to eat, you can go to the supermarket or the market to buy. You don't have to worry about buying a favorite food. Life is rich, and civilized diseases are quietly following. According to the survey, in the 1990s, about 1.6 million people in China suffered from cancer each year, and about 1.3 million people died of cancer each year. Compared with the 1970s, the number of cancers per year has increased by about 700,000. **As China's industrialization, urbanization and population aging process accelerates, if you do not pay attention to environmental protection, it will cause pollution of water, air and soil. The result is an increase in the number of substances in the food that are carcinogenic and mutagenic. There are major safety hazards in food. At the** same time, bad eating habits and unreasonable diet can also cause cancer, or promote the occurrence and development of cancer. Therefore, to eliminate the effects of carcinogens on people from food, it is necessary to actively prevent the occurrence of cancer.

Suggestions for diet preventing cancer

According to the experts' estimates, a diet containing a lot of vegetables and fruits (400-800g per person per day) can reduce more than 20% of all cancers. The following points for cancer prevention diets are as follows:

1). Pay attention to drinking water hygiene, drink activated carbon filtered tap water and qualified commercial drinking water.

2). Eat rough-processed wheat, rice, corn, barley, oats and rye, etc., with these as the main food (600~800g per person per day).

3). A large number of vegetables and fruits (400~800g per person per day), and there should be a variety of varieties.

4). Limit the intake of red meat (pig, beef, and mutton). Each person is below 80g per day. Use fish, poultry or non-domestic animals instead of red meat.

5). Eggs are an important source of protein. Each person is limited to 1 or 2 eggs per day to avoid excessive intake of cholesterol.

6). Milk is an important source of protein and calcium, at least 2 cups per person per day (250ml for a cup).

7). Soy or soy products should be eaten at least 30g per person per day (1~2 cups of soy milk per person per day).

8). Limit foods that contain more fat, especially foods that have more fat from animal sources. The edible vegetable oil should not exceed 2-3 tablespoons per person per day (mixed coconut oil, rapeseed oil, corn oil in a ratio of 1:1.5:1).

9). Adults should have less than 6g of salt per person per day. Eat less salted, salted fish and pickles.

10). Eat less sweets, limit the intake of refined sugar, should not exceed 10g per person per day.

11). Do not drink alcohol. If you drink alcohol, males should be under 2 cups for 1 day (1 cup of wine is defined as 250ml beer, 100ml wine, 25ml hard liquor or equivalent); women are under 1 cup.

12). Drinks should be based on green tea and drink at least 2 cups of green tea a day.

13). Chew slowly, the diet should be regularly quantified, do not eat hot food.

14). Do not eat moldy food, do not eat smoked, fried and grilled food.

15). Do not smoke or chew tobacco.

Cancer is preventable. The prevention method is to abandon some of the incorrect traditional concepts and to choose a scientific and rational lifestyle and to remove bad habits, and to improve the environmental conditions of work and residence, and carefully adjust the structure of the diet. Through the joint efforts of the whole society and all citizens, the prevention of cancer will definitely achieve remarkable results.

10. The recommendations of cancer prevention diet

First, Establish a prevention-oriented thinking or establish a thinking based on prevention

Cancer is largely a preventable disease. Improving diet, controlling weight, and strengthening physical activity can reduce the incidence of cancer by 30% to 40%. According to the current cancer incidence, about 3 to 4 million new cancer patients can be reduced every year. This number may reach 4-6 million by 2025, which is a considerable figure. In addition to saving lives, the source of resources saved is also considerable.

In middle-income countries, the cost of treatment for each cancer patient is between $2,000 and $11,000. Therefore, the practical method for dealing with cancer is prevention.

Preventing and treating cancer is the ultimate two strategies for controlling tumors. However, the prevention of cancer is fundamental, and the idea of "prevention first" is worthy of advocacy. According to the World Health Organization, about one-third of cancers are preventable, 1/3 of cancer can be cured and one third of cancer patients can prolong life. Through years of extensive epidemiological investigations and laboratory research, To date, at least 30 of the causes of cancer are known. As long as it can eliminate the known various carcinogenic factors or reduce it to a lower limit, or blocking the way it touches or invades the human body, then it is possible to prevent cancer from happening. Diet is closely related to cancer because people eat every day. About half of all cancers are related to diet. It is now known that some foods can cause cancer and other foods can prevent cancer. Improving diet is one aspect of many ways to prevent cancer,

We must implement prevention-oriented thinking into daily diet adjustment.

Second, how to prevent tumors

In addition to dietary regulation, according to our current understanding of cancer, cancer prevention generally has four aspects:

1. Pay attention to hygiene, enhance physical fitness, actively carry out physical exercise, and enhance physical fitness to prevent human aging, which is of great benefit to prevent cancer. Optimism, cheerfulness, carefreeness, and reduced mental stress are very helpful in improving human immunity and preventing tumors.

2. Eliminating or reducing the impact of carcinogenic factors and eliminating the effects of chemical, physical and biological carcinogenic factors on the human body from industrial and agricultural production, environmental sanitation, and living habits have positive significance for preventing tumors. Based on the understanding of tumor epidemiology and finding clues to the cause in some high-incidence areas, targeted preventive measures were put forward and received very good results.

3. Deal with precancerous lesions in time.

What is precancerous lesion?

Some diseases are not cancers themselves, but if they are not treated in time, they may develop into cancer on this basis.

For example, keratosis of the skin, hypertrophic scars, chronic ulcers, fistulas, leukoplakia of the skin and mucous membranes, black sputum that grows in areas susceptible to friction, and papilloma of the skin and mucous membranes; a polyp of rectum, colon and stomach, gastric ulcer, atrophic and hypertrophic gastritis; another example is cystic hyperplasia of the breast, breast fibroadenomas and intraductal papilloma of the breast; some patients with chronic hepatitis may develop cirrhosis. And cirrhosis has a close relationship with liver cancer;and also, cervical erosion, tearing, valgus, polyps; cryptorchidism or testicular insufficiency or testicular incomplete declining, foreskin is too long and phimosis.

It is required instructions that the precancerous lesions mentioned above do not necessarily become cancers. Even if a very small number of cancers occur, a longer course is also required. Therefore, early treatment can remove the condition of cancer and strive to eliminate security risks in the bud.

4. Prevention of cancer must pay attention to "three early", the so-called "three early" is early detection, early diagnosis and early treatment.

Cancer is not obvious in early symptoms, or similar to the symptoms of other diseases and is not easy to distinguish, so be vigilant and familiar with the early manifestations of common cancer. Early detection, early diagnosis and early treatment are very important. According to the specific situation in China, we believe that the following 10 symptoms deserve everyone's attention:

(1) A hard lump in any part of the body, such as the breast, neck or abdomen, especially faster;

(2) Any part of the body, such as the tongue, buccal mucosa, skin, etc., has no trauma and ulceration. Especially when it is not cured for a long time;

(3) Women with middle-aged or older have irregular vaginal bleeding or increased vaginal discharge;

(4) When eating, the sternum is swelled, burning, foreign body sensation or progressive aggravation of swallowing;

(5) a long-term cure for dry cough or sputum with blood;

(6) the long-term indigestion, progressive loss of appetite, weight loss. The stool is black, and no clear reason has been found;

(7) Changes in bowel habits, sometimes blood in the stool;

(8) nasal congestion, nosebleeds, unilateral headache or accompanied by double vision;

(9) The black mole suddenly increases or ruptures, bleeds, and the original hair falls off;

(10) There is blood in the urine, but there is no pain.

(4) Personal prevention of cancer

(Four)

Personal prevention of cancer

1. Pay attention to your lifestyle

General speaking, lifestyle refers to a person's habits of clothing, food, shelter, and behavior, and some behavioral hobbies, of which diet is the main factor. Its relationship with cancer has been described in detail. Here are some specific suggestions for your reference.

(1) Suggestions on eating habits

1) Eat low-fat cereals or whole grains, fresh fruits and fresh vegetables, as well as low-fat dairy products, poultry, fish, lean meat, and soy products. Do not or try to avoid eating smoked or moldy foods.

2) Regular exercise or exercise as much as you can, maintain normal weight, reduce excessive calorie intake, and prevent obesity.

3) Don't overdrink alcohol, don't drink hard alcohol every day.

4) drink more green tea, do not drink too much sugar and additives.

5) Eat less roast and fry food; do not use too much oil during cooking to avoid too much soot to inhale.

6) For the geographical area in which you are located and the type of work you are doing, especially those who have a certain cancer, you should supplement some special diets and essential ingredients. If you have a risk of developing lung cancer, you should eat more foods rich in vitamins A and C, and even supplement these vitamins and trace elements.

(2) Suggestions for the living room

For the vast majority of people, people spend about 80-90% of their time indoors, and spend more than 70% of their time in the family.

Therefore, the quality of the living environment and the degree of pollution are related to people's physical and mental health.

In recent years, scientists have found that indoor pollution is no less than outdoor, even more serious than outdoor. And it thinks that "family is a hotbed of cancer." Regardless of whether it is alarmist or overstated, in order to meet the requirements of cancer prevention, we propose the following:

1). People living in the basement and on the lower floors (1st to 3rd floors) should always pay attention to ventilation, because low-rise houses, especially the basement, can be polluted by radiation such as radon and radium released from the ground.

2). interior decoration has become fashionable in China. When using materials, less synthetic materials are used, and natural building materials are used. Because synthetic materials are mostly organic compounds, some raw materials are carcinogenic. In addition, according to the information, the plastic coated decorative material is superior to the embossed foamed wallpaper, because the former is coated with decorative materials to prevent the precipitation of certain radiation.

3). The kitchen should have good ventilation facilities.

According to the survey, 52% of lung squamous cell carcinoma and 61% of lung adenocarcinoma in the population are caused by kitchen oil fume pollution.

4). It is recommended to plant some flowers and plants indoors, which not only makes you indoors spring, but also adjusts the indoor oxygen concentration, especially the "grass flowers" such as cactus, and also releases a large amount of oxygen ions, which has the function of "negative ion generator". In addition, such as chrysanthemum, cyclamen, and beauty banana, there are adsorptions of carbon monoxide and harmful substances such as sulfur, fluorine and chlorine.

2. Advice on hobby behavior

Hobbies refer to people's special hobbies about certain things. One's hobbies belong to individual rights. However, many hobbies are not only harmful to oneself, but also harmful to the people around them and even to society. Therefore, it is necessary to speak out for certain hobbies. -------- "For the sake of you and your family and society," please abandon this behavior.

(1) The danger of smoking can be said to be "difficult to read bamboo", especially in the difficult relationship with lung cancer. Therefore, people must stop smoking, not to smoke in the home, in public places such as theaters, offices, conference rooms, restaurants, cars, etc. Smoking on this occasion is not only "harm yourself" but also "harming people". Passive smoking is more harmful to spouses and young children. Smoking can cause a higher incidence of spouse lung cancer, and the incidence of heart disease and high blood pressure in children is higher than that of non-smokers. In addition, there is information that if a mother smokes during pregnancy, her infant's chances of having a sudden infant death syndrome are significantly higher.

(2) Don't give people to respect by giving Tobacco, do not "eat respect", politely refuse to respect the smoke of which others give you, can be polite. "I am not good at scorpion, coughing, not smoking."

(3) Do not develop habits such as chewing tobacco or betel nut, this behavior is easy to cause oral cancer and lip cancer.

(4) Do not abuse drugs and strictly prohibit drug trafficking and drug abuse. Sharing syringes is one of the main ways to spread AIDS.

3. Protection against drugs and medical exposure

People often superstitious drugs, especially "tonic", that some drugs can not only cure diseases, but also improve health and prevent diseases. Nowadays, all kinds of supplement crystals are coming in from the rush or surging rushly, and it is not known that many "tonics" are lack of strict identification. And it is not known about whether they have "three-way" effect or not. As for certain drugs, it can damage the normal function of cells, causing DNA mutations and causing cancer.

Therefore, we propose the following recommendations for the use of drugs and radiation.

As for certain drugs, it can damage the normal function of cells, causing DNA mutations and causing cancer. Therefore, we propose the following recommendations for the use of drugs and radiation.

(1) Do not use hormones for a long time, such as diethylstilbestrol can cause cervical cancer, vaginal cancer and so on. Androgen plus 17 monomethyl substitutes can cause lung cancer.

(2) It is not possible to use certain anticancer drugs for a long time and inappropriately, such as alkylated anticancer drug nitrogen mustard can induce lymphoma, leukemia, etc.

(3) Do not abuse certain antibiotics, such as chloramphenicol, which can cause aplastic anemia. There are individual cases which therefore cause leukemia.

(4) Do not abuse hydantoin derivatives such as lenidine. It may be associated with malignant lymphoma; the depression drug phenisolide may be associated with the occurrence of Hodgkin's disease.

(5) Do not perform an X-ray examination or a dental x-ray examination if it is not necessary. For your own x-ray examination, you must have your own record so that you can refer to your doctor for medical treatment.

(6) There is information to prove that women underwent abdominal X-ray examinations during pregnancy, and the risk of leukemia in their children increased from 4 to 100 in every 100,000 people. Therefore, avoid exposing the abdomen when it is not necessary.

4. General medical advice

General medical care suggests that although it is not clearly targeted, it has an universal cancer prevention significance and has a certain effectiveness.

(1) Do not drink unclean river water or other polluted water.

A lot of data show that there are many carcinogenic factors in unclean water, such as various molds, bacteria pollution, and carcinogens such as nitrosamines and aflatoxins.

(2) Pay attention to the prevention of hepatitis B and hepatitis C, especially the latter often causes cirrhosis, which eventually leads to the formation of liver cancer.

(3) Prevention of parasitic infections.

Some parasitic infections are associated with certain cancers. For example, infection with Clonorchis sinensis is associated with liver cancer and cholangiocarcinoma; schistosomiasis infection is associated with liver cancer and colorectal cancer.

(4) Pay attention to oral hygiene.

Brushing your teeth every day helps prevent oral cancer and gum cancer.

(5) Familiar with the medical knowledge of certain precancerous lesions and genetic diseases, in order to be vigilant against them, and conduct regular inspections to achieve "preventing problems before they occur", such as familial colon polyposis, xeroderma pigmentosum, mucosal leukoplakia and the like.

(6) For certain chronic inflammations, such as cervicitis, as well as chronic ulcer disease. It is necessary to treat and follow up in time to prevent deterioration.

(7) Pay attention to physical exercise and enhance disease resistance, especially immunity.

(8) Keep the "state of mind" safe. The state of mind mentioned here refers to a weak and lasting emotional state. Don't restrain yourself excessively, suppress anger and too much dissatisfaction and insecurity.

These factors may affect the occurrence and development of cancer more or less. Maintaining the "state of mind" of Enron or peace or calm.

In the above aspects, perhaps it can be representative to precautionary measures taken at present to people's understanding of the causes of cancer. It is believed that with the deeper understanding of cancer, more effective preventive measures can be adopted. For everyone, the premise is to understand the knowledge about cancer, and to eliminate the carcinogenic factors in the environment, to benefit human beings, and to protect themselves.

(5) Self-early discovery of cancer

(1) Suspected symptoms of early cancer

The difficulty in early diagnosis of cancer is that it often lacks symptoms early, or has symptoms that are not specific. Once there are more obvious symptoms, the cancer may have been going on for a while, and the mass at this time is often more than 1 cm in diameter. Of course, the likelihood of healing at this time is much smaller than that of smaller tumors. Therefore, if a person has a deep understanding of his body and is alert to cancer, it is not that it is impossible to find an earlier cancer. Below, we draw attention to the following symptoms or manifestations, perhaps they are the clues and early signs of cancer.

1. Significant weight loss

A healthy person can maintain relative stability without special reasons. Even with weight loss, it is often the obvious reason to check.

However, if a person's "unexplained" weight loss, especially in a short period of time, such as a drop of 5 kg or more in a few months, it may be the first sign of cancer. This is more common in digestive tract tumors such as gastric cancer, pancreatic cancer, esophageal cancer, liver cancer, and lung cancer. It is also found in Hodgkin's disease and 'renal cell cancer. Therefore, weight loss for unknown reasons must not be taken lightly.

2. "unknown cause" fever

There are many diseases that cause fever, such as inflammation, rheumatism, etc. Therefore, it is often ignored by doctors or individuals, but fever is also one of the common symptoms of cancer patients. Cancer fever may be caused by cancer cell death, and may also be associated with infection. This is more common in Hodgkin's disease, non-Hodgkin's lymphoma, chronic leukemia, atrial myxoma, and renal cell carcinoma.

3. Tired and weak

This is also a symptom of atypical cancer. People who are middle-aged are often physically weak because of their busy work, so many people are tired all day long. However, if fatigue is too difficult to recover and shows weakness, you must be vigilant. It often suggests that a certain part of the human body may have hidden dangers, such as stomach cancer, colon cancer, and Hodgkin's disease.

4. Pain

Tumors are painless neoplasms, but here are the early stages of cancer. Once the cancer is advanced, there is more pain, the so-called "cancerous pain", and the patient is unbearable. However, sometimes there are some special types of pain that help to detect curable malignancies. Therefore, it is not sloppy or ignore for pain.

5. Cough

Men, women, and children often suffer from coughs, especially during the fall and winter seasons, so people are more accustomed to it. However, we want to point out that "the more than forty years, the long-term cough", you must think about the possibility of lung cancer, especially those with a history of serious smoking and family history of lung cancer cannot be taken lightly.

6. Stool and nature change

Most people have good bowel habits, one time a day, or once a day. Generally, the nature of stool is also relatively constant. However, if the number of stools, the nature has changed, or the stool becomes thinner or even unreasonable, the use of laxatives is not good, even those with bloody stools must be carefully examined.

This is especially important for those who are older, or have a family history of colon cancer or a history of schistosomiasis.

7. Chronic ulcer

Prolonged healing skin ulcers, to consider the possibility of basal cell carcinoma or squamous cell carcinoma, should be excised and sent to biopsy. Chronic cervicitis, cervical erosion should often be done vaginal smear, and even biopsy; chronic oral ulcers should be closely watched and biopsy should be performed if necessary, especially for severe smokers, alcoholics, and chewing tobacco and betel nut. For chronic gastric ulcers, especially atrophic gastritis, frequent follow-up is also required.

8. Bleeding

Small and persistent bleeding, especially in certain areas, is highly vigilant, and blood in the stool is an early sign of colorectal cancer.

9. hard to swallow

Dysphagia, especially progressive, that is, difficulty in swallowing coarse foods at first, followed by difficulty in swallowing soft foods, it is necessary to think of esophageal cancer, especially in some high-incidence areas.

10. hoarse voice

Long-term hoarseness caused by non-inflammation or local strain, suggesting laryngeal or lung cancer and thyroid cancer, should be used for laryngoscopy or X-ray examination.

11. Activity change of wart versus mole

Wart and mole are very common, almost everyone has several. But if they suddenly cause a feeling of pain, itching, or a faster growth rate or a different pigment, don't care.

12. Touching mass

The mass may be a benign tumor, such as a lipoma, or it may be a thickening of local tissue, or it may be an inflammatory reaction followed by fibrosis. However, once the texture and growth rate have changed, a biopsy is required.

(2) The World Health Organization has issued eight warning signals as a reference for early signs of cancer.

As shown below or the following figures:

World Health Organization proposes eight warning signs as a reference for early cancer signs.

a. The touched hard nodule or firm area in thyroid, breast, skin or tongue

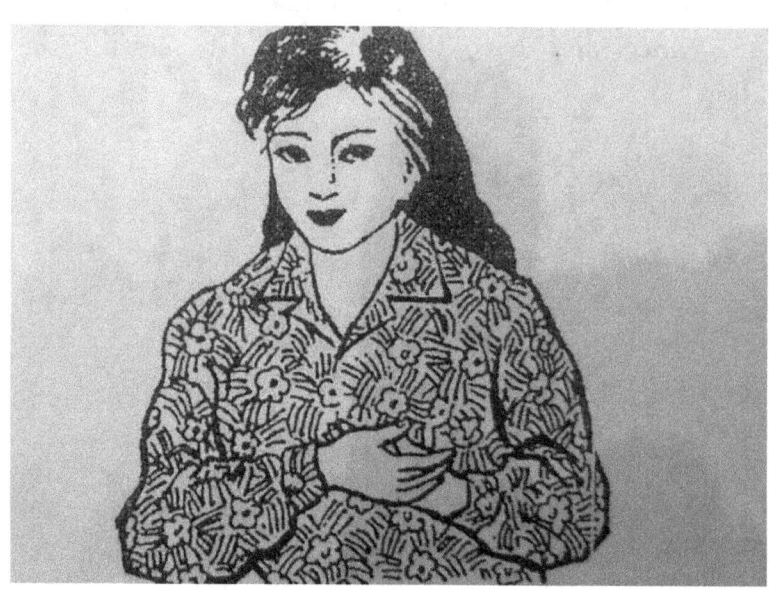

b. The mole suddenly and significantly changes

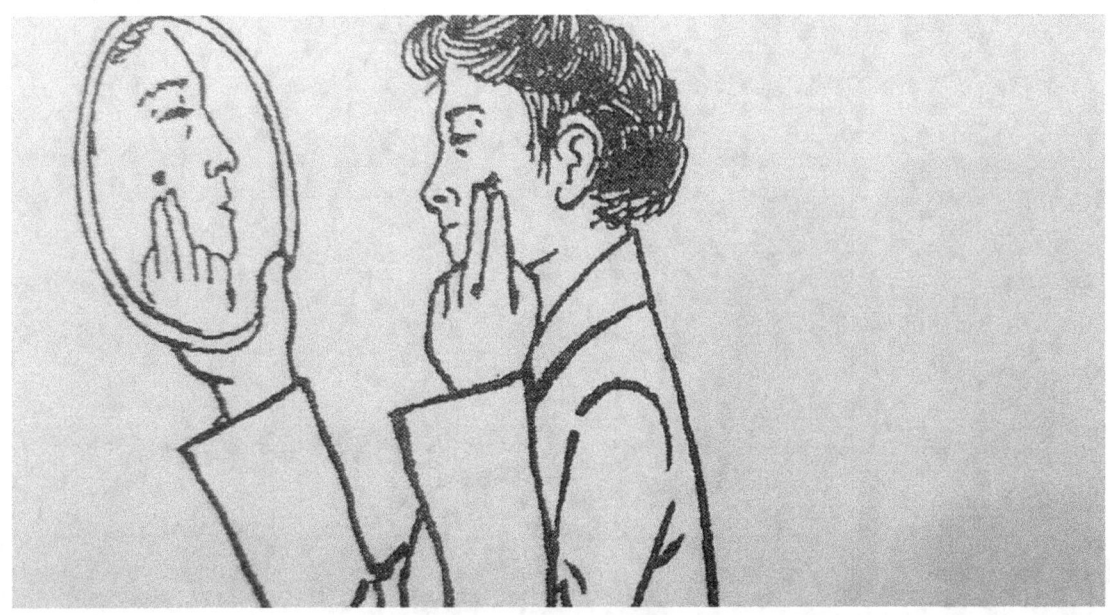

c. The long-term indigestion without reason

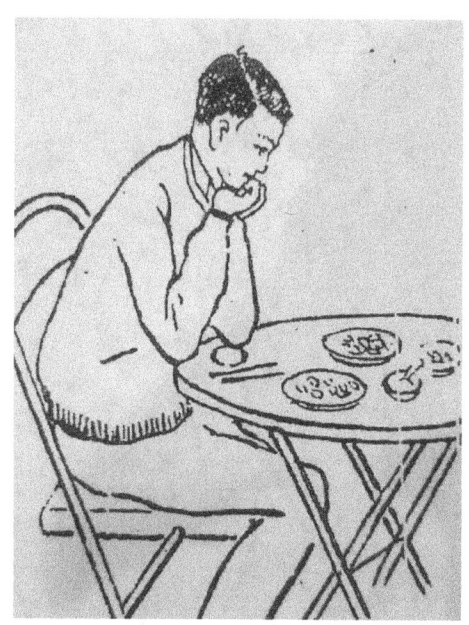

d. The lasting hoarse voice and dry cough and difficult swallow

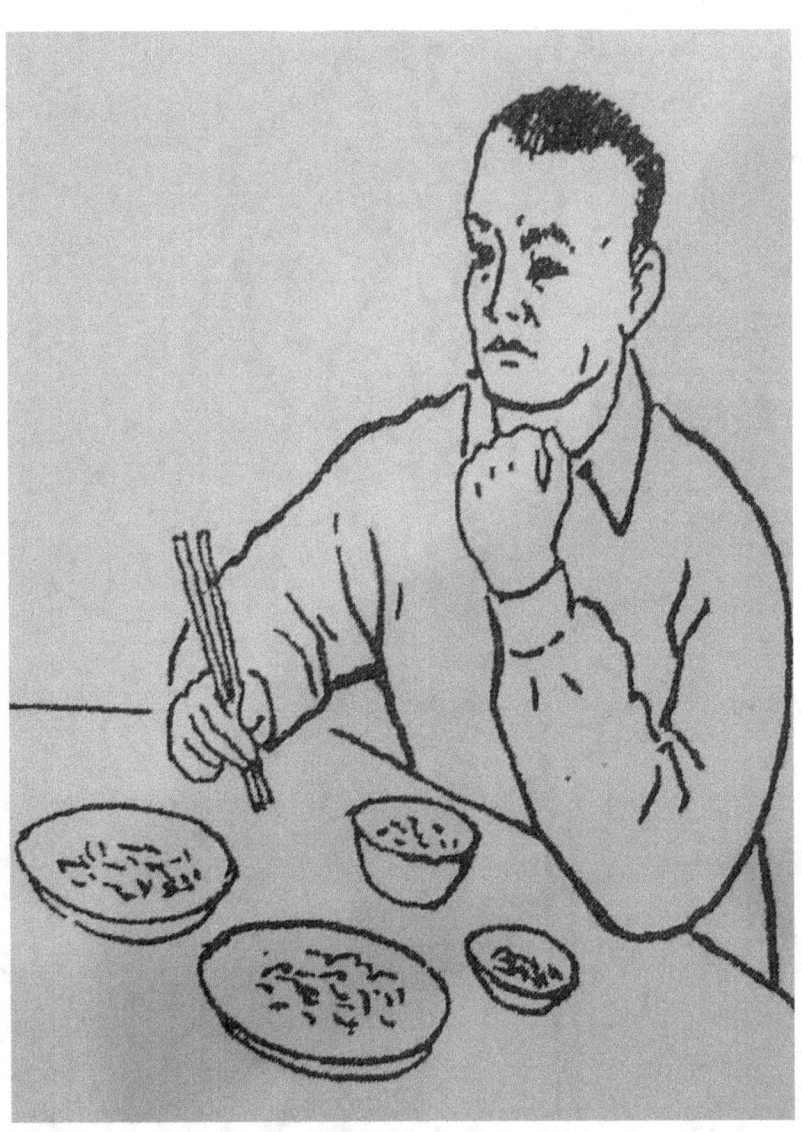

e. The irregular period with huge bleeding or the bleeding outside the period

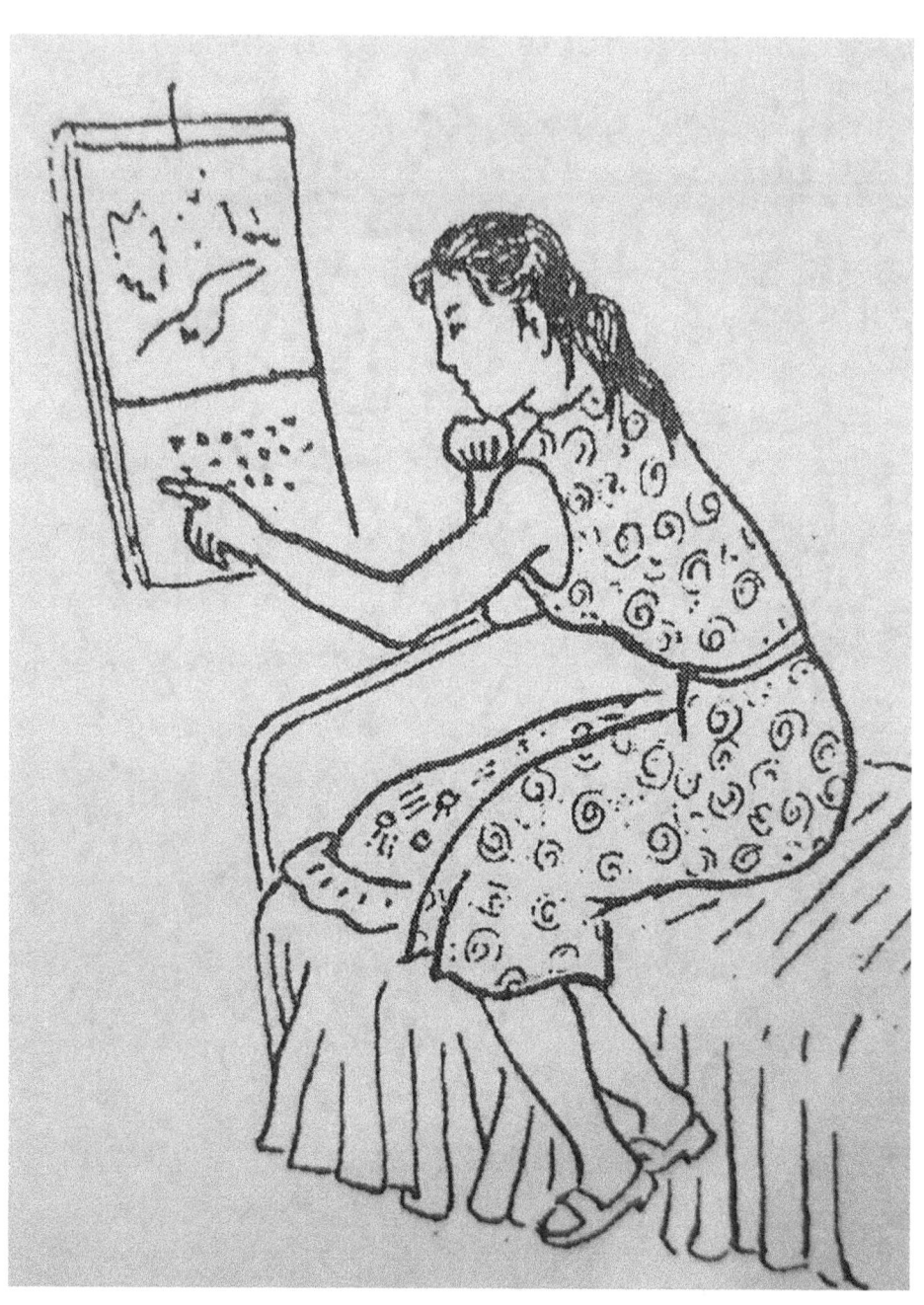

f. The blood urine and stool and nose bleeding or ear bleeding

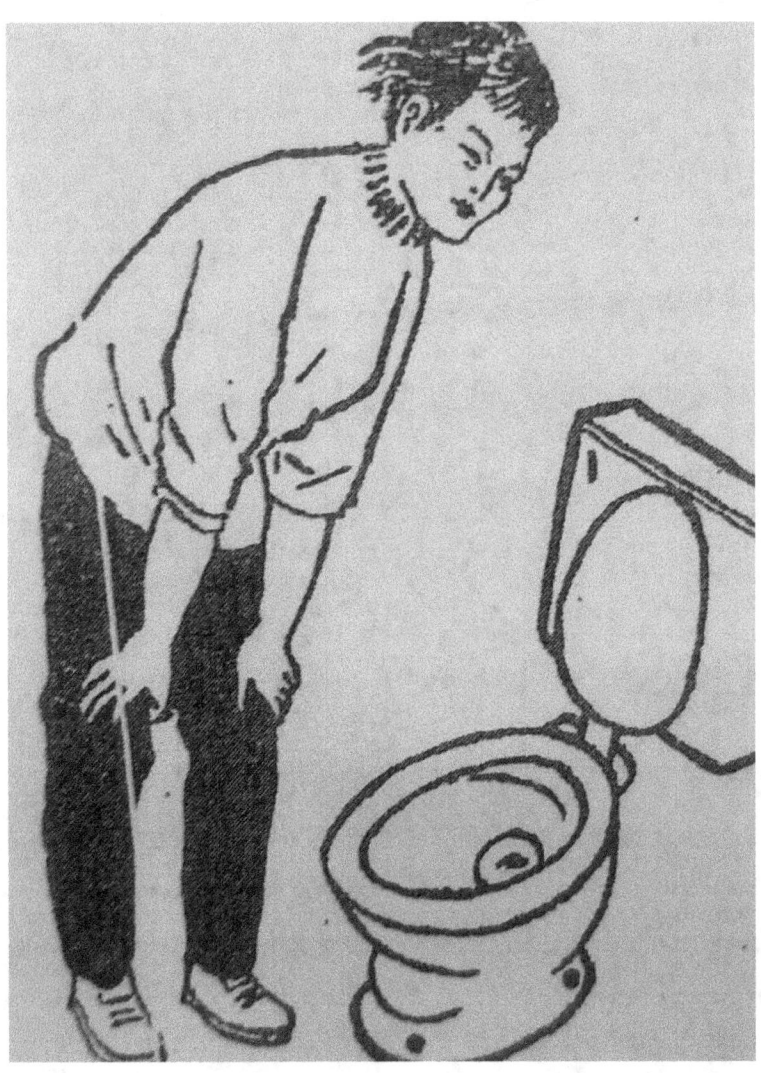

G. The lasting and no recovery wound and ulcer and the lump without disappearing

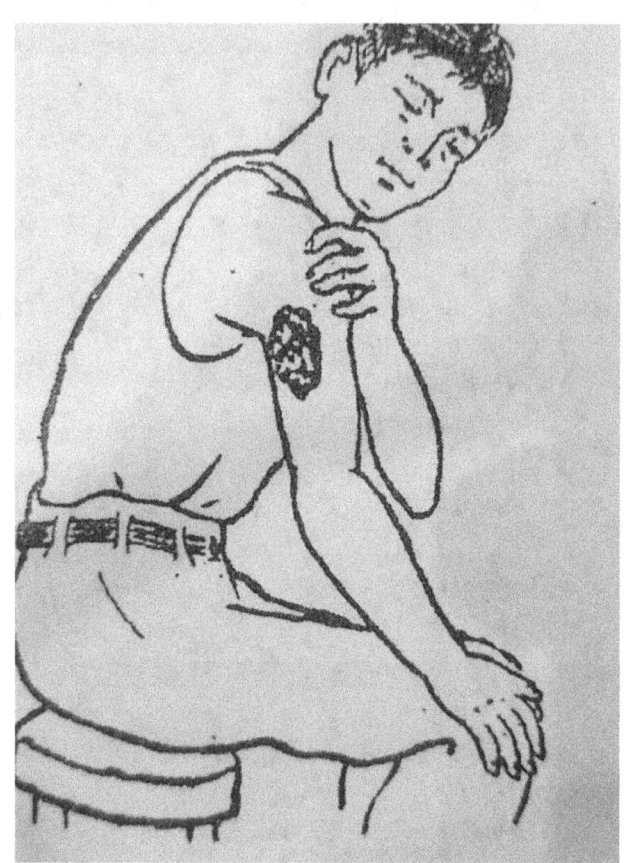

h. The weight loss without reasons

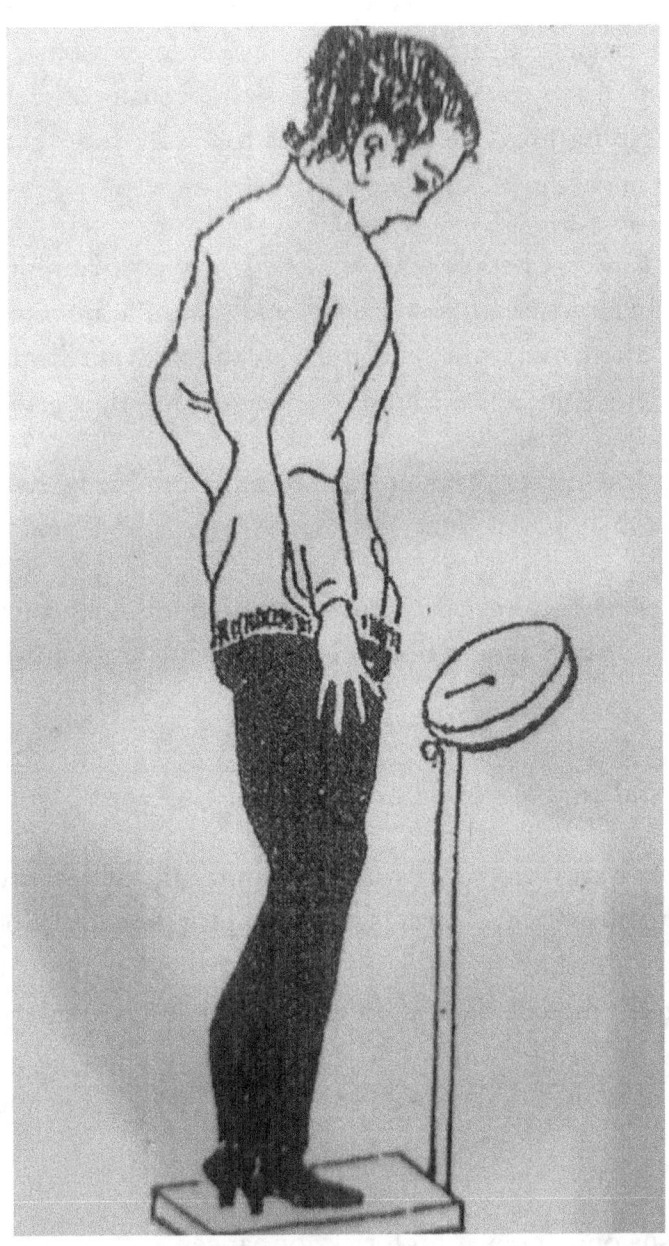

(6) Census of cancer in the 21st century

(Six)

21st Century Cancer Census

The importance of the cancer census has been detailed in the previous chapters of this book, but the census requires people to have at least a basic knowledge about cancer; have a team of the well-trained professional census officer. There must be a certain economic strength. More important is to create some simple and accurate census techniques or methods.

In fact, in the last century, people have achieved very gratifying results in the early diagnosis of cervical cancer. In some developed countries, women regularly take cervical smear on their own and send them to the relevant health care center for examination. Therefore, it can be found in time whether the cervix is malignant.

In addition to cervical cancer, women learn to self-examine breasts and also reduce breast cancer mortality.

However, for most cancers, the census is not so simple. For this reason, in the 21st century, human beings will certainly make efforts in the following areas and benefit from it.

1. Establish a global cancer surveillance system

Mastering the cancer and related trends of carcinogenic factors and formulating the scientific basis for cancer control strategies, the International Oncology Registration Association was established in 1965, and standardized statistical indicators were formulated to publish disease data on five continents on a regular basis. Facts have proved that global unified planning and multi-party monitoring are very beneficial for humans to avoid or deal with those carcinogenic risk factors and eliminate them.

2. Focus the census on people at high risk for cancer

Although the life and medical care of all human beings will be improved in the 21st century, it is necessary to conduct a census of certain procedures among billions of people. On the one hand, it is a huge economic burden, and on the other hand, it may not be necessary.

To this end, pay full attention to those who have a high risk of cancer, like some tumors with genetic predisposition, such as childhood retinoblastoma, Familial multiple colonic polyposis, patients with pigmented dry skin disease or there are special carcinogenic factors (such as radiation) exposed. Only in this way can we get twice the result with half the effort.

3. Looking for more specific census means

With the development of molecular biology, molecular epidemiology and other disciplines, people will find more accurate and simple census means. It is expected that in the 21st century, people will find more specific cancer cells or products of oncogenes. For example, cancer cell surface antigens, as well as the tumor suppressor gene P53 protein, can greatly advance the diagnosis of cancer.

(7) Prevention of cancer in the 21st century

(Seven)

Cancer prevention in the 21st century

There are big differences of the incidence of most cancers between countries and regions, therefore, cancer is thought to be mainly caused by factors such as the environment, diet, and hobbies. Therefore, in the 21st century, people will attach great importance to carcinogenic factors in the environment and strive to eliminate them.

1. Smoke-free world

With people's awareness of the dangers of smoking(regardless of personal, family, and socio-economic development), it is knowing that it is "a hundred harms and no benefit". In the years to come, it is bound to "Yuyu clarify Wan Lie", the whole world will be a smoke-free world. Optimistic scientists believe that this bad habit will never last until the middle of the 21st century. Of course, by then, lung cancer, esophageal cancer, bladder cancer, laryngeal cancer, lip cancer and oral cancer will definitely decline or drastically reduced.

2. People are no longer obese

Doctors have long discovered that colorectal cancer and breast cancer are more common in economically developed countries, and this has a certain relationship with high-fat diets.

People should realize that "the brain is full of fat," it is not a "blessing", but a "yellow card" for good health.

People in the 21st century will surely get more scientific medical guidance and can lose weight in terms of reasonable diet and proper exercise. It is no longer obese, and can keep the mouth shut in order to prevent "disease (cancer) from the mouth."

3. Anticipation and elimination of carcinogenic factors

This is a difficult task because the carcinogen is the objective existence of the world. Some are staying in the same place as celestial bodies, such as ultraviolet rays, earth rays, radioactive elements, etc.;

Some are staying in the same place as the human body, such as various hormones, and even certain nutrients such as tryptophan. But more importantly, in human production activities, thousands of carcinogenic factors, such as certain insecticides, herbicides, artificial rubber and plastics, drugs, etc., are constantly being produced. However, the detection of carcinogenicity of these substances is extremely difficult. On the one hand, it is a large number. On the one hand, it is costly and time-consuming, and it will make people unable to do anything.

Therefore, in the 21st century, people strive to find a way to predict the carcinogenicity of a substance, and the experiment to detect carcinogenesis is simple, accurate and economical.

4. XZ-C proposes that in order to overcome cancer and to launch the general attack of cancer, it must establish the Environmental Protection Cancer Research Institute and carry out the cancer prevention system project to open a new era of cancer prevention research and cancer prevention system engineering in the 21st century.

In the search for the cause and condition of cancer, it is remarkable that it is found that more than 90% of cancers are caused by environmental factors.

The Cancer Research Institute should conduct cancer prevention research to find cancer-causing factors, detect damage to humans caused by carcinogens or carcinogenic factors, and trace the source of carcinogens or carcinogenic factors, and to study how to reduce or prevent these carcinogens.

5. How to overcome cancer? How to prevent cancer?

XZ-C proposed: "Creating the Environmental Protection and Health Cancer Prevention Research Institute" to carry out cancer prevention system engineering and establish a high-level laboratory.

XZ-C proposes:

Dawning A type anti-cancer plan

Dawning B type anti-cancer plan

Dawning D-type anti-cancer plan

Because cancer patients cover the whole world, the pollution of industrial and agricultural wastewater and waste residue and waste gas also cover the whole world, It is imperative that the global effort be made to overcome cancer and to launch the general attack on cancer, to study these sources of pollution, and to try to stop at the source and to strive to eliminate security risks in the bud.

www.ingramcontent.com/pod-product-compliance
Lightning Source LLC
Chambersburg PA
CBHW062320220526
45469CB00008B/2579